An Integrative Medicine Approach to **Modern Eye Care**

An Integrative Medicine Approach to **Modern Eye Care**

Alfred Anduze, MD
John C. Merritt, MD

TATE PUBLISHING
AND ENTERPRISES, LLC

Published by Tate Publishing & Enterprises, LLC
127 E. Trade Center Terrace | Mustang, Oklahoma 73064 USA
1.888.361.9473 | www.tatepublishing.com

Tate Publishing is committed to excellence in the publishing industry. The company reflects the philosophy established by the founders, based on Psalm 68:11,
"The Lord gave the word and great was the company of those who published it."

Cover design by Jim Villaflores
Interior design by Jomar Ouano

Published in the United States of America

ISBN: 978-1-63063-273-1
1. Medical / Optometry
2. Medical / Holistic Medicine
14.03.07

Dedication

This book is dedicated to the faculty and staff at the University of Arizona, Tucson School of Integrative Medicine and my classmates and colleagues in the vibrant field of integrative medicine the world over.

And especially to Drs. Andrew Weil, Victoria Maizes, Tieraona Lowdog, Randy Horowitz, Howard Silverman, for their inspiration, knowledge, and good example.

And to my wife, Sari, whose idea was to pursue this course and persist in establishing a foundation for the much-needed change direction of medicine and for becoming a part of the integrative medicine family.

Acknowledgments

Thank you to Dr. Tieraona Low Dog for the introduction, inspiration, and encouragement to get this book organized and into print.

Photographs in chapter six designated with * are from Wikipedia and Google free access.

All other photographs are by the author.

We would like to express a special gratitude to the editor, Selena Anduze-Anaya, whose knowledge and expertise in the field of natural health was a great contribution to this work.

Thank you to Dr. Andrew Weil for bringing integrative medicine into the forefront of health care education. It is a tough battle, but we are winning.

Contents

Foreword

When I was asked to write the foreword for this book, I was startled to review some of the statistics about the state of eye health in the United States. According to the American Academy of Ophthalmology, by the age of eighty, more than half of all Americans have cataracts and more than two million Americans over the age of fifty have advanced macular degeneration, the stage most likely to cause severe vision impairment. Diabetes now affects more than 11 percent of all adults over the age of twenty. The longer someone has diabetes, the greater the risk for developing diabetic retinopathy, another leading cause of blindness in the United States. Roughly, one out of three Americans are nearsighted. While nearsightedness is in part due to genetics, there is evidence that too much close work is a contributing factor. We spend an inordinate amount of time staring at blackboards, cell phones, and computer screens; and not enough time outdoors looking at distant objects to keep the muscles that control distant vision strong and flexible.

As the founder and director of the University of Arizona Center for Integrative Medicine, I have devoted most of my career to training health care practitioners in integrative medicine. This discipline is healing-oriented medicine that takes account of the whole person (body, mind, and spirit), including all aspects of lifestyle. It emphasizes the therapeutic relationship and makes use of all appropriate therapies, both conventional and alternative.

Integrative medicine selects the very best, scientifically validated therapies from conventional, complementary, and alternative systems. From the role of diet and exercise in preventing diabetes to the research showing that certain antioxidants and fish oil can prevent the progression of age-related macular degeneration, there is no doubt that integrative approaches have a place in modern-day ophthalmology.

This is why I am delighted that Alfred Anduze, MD, one of only a handful of ophthalmologists in the world to complete our Center's Fellowship in Integrative Medicine, and John Merritt, MD, have written *An Integrative Medicine Approach to Modern Eye Care*. I highly recommend it.

—Andrew Weil, MD
Tucson, Arizona, USA
September 2012

Preface

An integrative medicine approach to modern eye care is needed because eye diseases can range in causes from genetics, environmental toxins, free radicals, severe oxidative stress, decreased immunity, age, inflammation, degeneration, decreased circulation, chronic dehydration, lack of adequate physical activity, inadequate rest, to even our current treatments. Pharmaceutical drugs are often toxic and our surgical procedures may sometimes be more detrimental than beneficial. Despite great technological advances in cataract surgery, very little has been done to prevent cataracts. No matter how wonderful, an artificially manufactured multifocal intraocular lens is never the same as a DNA-created crystalline one, so why not keep your natural lens and still see well into your nineties.

This book provides some answers to the patient question, "What else can be done other than drugs or surgery to preserve my eyesight?"

Ophthalmology, along with internal and family medicine, has failed to control or even reduce the incidence of and rising population for disabilities, due to conditions such as diabetes, hypertension, glaucoma, and macular degeneration. The incidence and prevalence continue to rise.

There are many factors that determine why one 68-year-old person develops debilitating cataracts and another does not. A great deal of my time and energy has been spent in trying to impart this concept to my colleagues, some of whom remain skeptical. The patients' socioeconomic status, immediate environment, emotional state, family and social history, nutritional habits, and sedentary lifestyles all play a role in the outcome of their treatment and recovery regimens. The majority of poor outcomes in eye disease are a direct result of chronic inflammation and/or poor circulation. Modern treatment methods via steroids, antibiotics, and antimetabolites are directed at symptoms and often spare underlying causes. They may even be involved in the creation of *new diseases* for which more drugs are created. These chronic progressive conditions involve the entire body and should be addressed through attention to the patient as a whole. Lifestyle changes that target general health and also include both the conventional and traditional medical approach are well worth the effort at prevention and cure.

Considering case scenarios, a 45-year-old female accompanies her mother, who is wheelchair bound and is 73 years old and suffers from obesity, arthritis, diabetes, hypertension, and reduced vision due to cataracts, glaucoma, and macular degeneration. The daughter asks the physician how he/she can prevent such debilitations from happening to her.

In a second-case scenario, a 60-year-old male with +1 lens sclerosis on slit lamp exam and 20/25 best corrected vision asks for ways to prevent his cataract from advancing.

In a third-case scenario, a 40-year-old male with an Afro-Caribbean ancestry, a family history of blindness from glaucoma, and borderline intraocular pressures of 19 and 21 mmHg, asks if he can use medical marijuana.

With all of the patients mentioned above, a discussion on an Integrative Approach to Eye Care is in order. Each individual is offered specific protocols of preventive strategies. These include selective and appropriate dietary regimen, possible use of botanicals, specific physical activity, mind-body stress control, energy medicine, homeopathy, Chinese and Ayurvedic therapies, and guidance to lifestyle changes best suited to their conditions. The risks and benefits of each modality should be weighed in relation to and conjunction with those of conventional therapies. One is not intended to replace the other. In the age of the Internet and with the resurgence of *alternative medicine*, patients can acquire information about vitamins and supplements, but perhaps not the appropriate applications, dosages, combinations, and side effects. Research is closely linked to advertising and all claims may not always be accurate.

Continuation of poor health remains a problem. This is due in part to inadequate access of a large part of our population to health care, doctors' neglect of preventive measures, overpriced or unavailable pharmaceuticals, bad insurance practices rooted in profit motives, and relentless misleading in advertising. Arrogance and continued preoccupation with diagnostics and use of exorbitant, dangerous treatments often encourage patients' distrust of the system. Meanwhile, the population grows fatter and weaker.

> Our way of life is killing us. Risky behavior and the practices associated with modern living account for roughly half of premature deaths in the USA. Although patients' visits and expenditures to alternative medical practitioners are eclipsing those to conventional practitioners, the medical profession has taken little notice, especially ophthalmologists. We are still preoccupied with the latest and most precise lasers, magnetic imaging machines, strongest blocking drugs, and sharpest scalpels. Our attitudes are stuck on quantity instead of quality. The patient who has had five procedures for cataract, glaucoma, and retinal detachment and who has barely 20/400 vision is applauded as having undergone heroic successful treatment, while the causes of his or her condition are largely ignored. How did he/she get this way in the first place? The answer usually lies in the inappropriate lifestyle choices of the patients, which are additionally passed over

> or given very little attention by their doctors. For many, without a scalpel and the prescription pad, there is nothing left to offer. By exploring and paying attention to the interconnections of lifestyle and disease, one can hope to reduce one with the benefits of the other. "It is much more important to know what sort of patient has the disease than what sort of disease the patient has."
>
> —Sir William Osler, MD

> "The health status of the body and the mind has everything to do with the presence of disease, progression and outcome of the eye."
>
> —Alfred Anduze, MD

In a brief synopsis, the first chapter examines the effects of time and lifestyle on the tissues of the eye with the goal being to reduce the risk of eye disease and improve the quality of life. Why do some people age better than others? It is no secret that maintaining basic good health is a key in preserving the body and especially the senses. One cannot stop aging, but one can influence the process. For example, inflammation is a major cause of eye disease. The recognition and reduction of preop inflammation and promotion of post-op healing should be the focus of all interventional eye care. That would mean less reliance on steroids and antibiotics and more attention paid to the basic principles of natural healing. A healthy person will heal better than a sick one. Control of inflammation is the key to prevention of disease and achievement of successful outcomes. This concept will be repeated and applied throughout the remaining chapters.

Toxins in both our food and environment play a huge role in today's degenerative and neurological disorders. They promote inflammation, tissue destruction, and loss of function. Detoxification has a positive influence on eye disease. The causes of many eye disorders such as cataracts, glaucoma, diabetic eye disease, macular degeneration, optic nerve, and other disorders can be linked to other concomitant internal diseases. These, in turn, are linked to basic lifestyle functions such as lack of exercise, inadequate rest, poor circulation, poor elimination, and generalized malaise. Nutrition is of the utmost importance. Bad food choices lead to an accumulation of omega-6 and the dispensation of free radicals, which damage body tissues. Weight control is an asset when dealing with chronic diseases. The benefits of antioxidants in whole food far outweigh the risks of pharmaceuticals. Stress, a direct cause of abnormal release of cortisol, has detrimental effects on the body, especially on highly specialized organs like the eyes. Lack of exercise leads to small-vessel dysfunction and poor blood perfusion. This is crucial in glaucoma management. Botanicals offer a wide range of remedies and anti-inflammation treatments, but caution must be advised in regard to inadequate preparation, misleading claims, and watchfulness with poisonous plant parts. The roles of energy medicine, homeopathy, and Chinese and Ayurvedic medicine are less well defined but will be discussed with respect to their contribution and application to eye care.

Though most persons of Caribbean descent are proud to acknowledge the success of traditional medicine, they still consider allopathic medicine as the norm and therefore somehow better. They are, however, eager to accept the possibilities of natural health and pursue protocols in preventive medicine for cataract, glaucoma management, retino-degenerative disease, and inflammation control that will promote general health rather than embrace surgery and drugs too readily.

This book is intended for ophthalmic residents, practicing ophthalmologists, academicians, and all medical personnel with an interest in prevention of disease and complete eye care. It is an attempt to provide answers to basic questions that deal not with alternative, but complimentary evidence-based therapies available to achieve the best clinical outcome.

It is the physicians' responsibility to promote good health, provide accurate information and a complete range of viable options, and to work with the patient as a partner with the goal of well being firmly in mind. If we do not accomplish this, we will soon become the *alternative*.

—Alfred L. Anduze, MD

Introduction

Leonardo Da Vinci once said, "The eye is the window of the human body through which it feels its way and enjoys the beauty of the world." Humans are highly visual creatures, devoting more of our brain to sight than any other sense. Poets and musicians have tried to capture the power of our eyes to convey and perceive emotion. The saying "A picture is worth a thousand words" speaks to the power of a painting, sculpture, face, or landscape to move us beyond words. It is imperative that we protect and preserve our eyesight, as our vision so dramatically impacts our sense of well-being.

While we generally associate poor lifestyle choices with heart disease, diabetes, and cancer, there is a growing body of data that suggests that these same choices can adversely impact our eyes. While most people know they should wear sunglasses and get regular exams, many are not aware of the impact of a poor diet on their vision. Diets rich in processed foods and low in fruits, vegetables, nuts, seeds, and fish can result in inadequate intake of nutrients vital to eye health. Studies conducted by the National Eye Institute have shown that vitamins C and E, beta-carotene, zinc, and copper can reduce the risk of developing age-related macular degeneration (AMD), a leading cause of vision loss in people over the age of sixty-five years. Intense research is now underway examining the protective effects of fish oil, lutein, and zeaxanthin, as recent evidence has shown that they slow the progress of AMD. Fish oil has also been shown to improve dry eye syndrome.

More than 60 percent of the American population is now overweight or obese, putting them at high risk for many chronic diseases, including blindness. In 2011, according to the Centers for Disease Control, 11 percent of American adults had diabetes and estimated that if trends continue, one in three adults will have the disease by 2050. Diabetic retinopathy is a leading cause of blindness in the United States. Diabetics also have double risk of glaucoma, the second leading cause of blindness. These data are particularly alarming and disappointing, given that a healthy diet, exercise, and weight management dramatically reduces the risk of diabetes, and thus, vision loss.

Given the epidemic of lifestyle-related chronic disease, one would expect physicians to be well-trained in how to motivate and counsel patients to eat a healthy diet, stop smoking, lose weight, or change other unhealthy behaviors. However, most physicians receive less than the twenty-five hours of nutrition education and even less about the role of vitamins and minerals in health. Integrative medicine is attempting to correct that deficit by teaching clinicians evidence-based approaches to health that takes into account the whole person, including all aspects of lifestyle.

As the fellowship director at the University of Arizona Center for Integrative Medicine, I was absolutely delighted to read *Integrative Medicine Approach to Modern Eye Care*. This book, the first of its kind, is an evidence-based roadmap for how integrative medicine can be employed to optimize eye health. Dr. Alfred Anduze, one of the only ophthalmologists in the world to have graduated from our 2-year, 1000-hour fellowship training program, is a true leader in this field. He is joined by Dr. John Merritt, professor of ophthalmology, who provided invaluable information from his experiences and early publications on natural medications for chronic eye diseases.

Patients need to understand the effects of lifestyle choices, the influence of diet on disease risk, the importance of regular physical activity, when and how to use preventive medical services, when to seek help from conventional doctors, and when natural remedies may be appropriate. This book more than answers those needs. Drs. Anduze and Merritt are highly trustworthy sources of information. This book is an important contribution to the fields of both integrative medicine and ophthalmology. I highly recommend it.

—Tieraona Low Dog, MD
Fellowship Director, Arizona Center
for Integrative Medicine
Clinical Associate Professor of Medicine,
University of Arizona College of Medicine
Chair: United States Pharmacopeia Dietary
Supplements Expert Panel, Safety
Author: *National Geographic's Life is Your Best Medicine*

Features and Preview of Goals

1. The principles of integrative medicine as applied to eye care, are to examine and treat the whole person, including emotional, mental, physical, and spiritual health.
2. Strive for prevention and control of inflammation with attention to enhancement of the immune system.
3. Promote natural wound healing with less use of steroids and antibiotics for routine external trauma and surgeries.
4. Pay strict attention to proper and appropriate basic nutrition, with attention to elimination, toxicity, and weight control.
5. Highlight the efficacy of botanicals in the treatment of eye conditions, including marijuana and exercise for glaucoma, cataract prevention and possible reversal, control of inflammation and prevention, and alleviation of degenerative diseases.
6. Promote regular exercise to increase blood perfusion, reduce stress, improve vital signs, and enhance immunity.
7. Minimize strong drug and surgical interventions.
8. Control physical and emotional stress through comprehension and mind-body therapies.
9. Benefits of eastern Medicine disciplines in promotion of eye health.

10. Achievement of well-being and good health.
11. A healthy body will translate into healthy eyes and good eyesight.

Complimentary Medical Therapies with Positive Evidence-based Studies:

1. Acupuncture
2. Alexander technique
3. Aromatherapy
4. Autogenic therapy
5. Ayurvedic
6. Biofeedback
7. Color therapy
8. Herbal medicine
9. Homeopathy
10. Hypnosis
11. Magnet therapy
12. Massage
13. Meditation
14. Naturopathy

—Alfred L. Anduze, MD, MH
Integrative Medicine

The Aging Eye: External Diseases

Case Scenario One:An 88-year-old female sits in a wheelchair in your waiting room. She is frail, has a sad countenance, and is wearing heavy clothing though we are located in the tropics. She suffers from multiple inflammatory conditions (arthritis, osteoporosis) and she has 20/400 vision due to bilateral nonglaucomatous optic atrophy. Mature nuclear sclerotic cataracts, entropia of the lower lids, blepharochalasis of the upper lids, degenerative corneal pterygia, and band keratopathy are among her conditions. She is accompanied by her friend, an 87-year-old female, who is pushing the wheelchair. The friend has 20/30 vision bilaterally, fairly normal adnexae, mild lens sclerosis +1, a cup/disc ratio of 0.3 and healthy retinal vasculature. Why?

"Proper aging makes a good rum great."

—Anonymous

Eye Signs of Aging: Droopy eyelids, dermatochalasis, blepharochalasis, chronic blepharitis, ptosis, facial wrinkles, papillomata, abnormal pigmentation, basal cell carcinoma, degenerative pingueculum and pterygium, squamous cell carcinoma, corneal thinning, arcus senilis, dark circles, dry eyes, epiphora, puffy eyes, chronic conjunctivitis, herpes zoster ophthalmicus, ectropion, entropion, glaucoma, cataract, floaters, retinal degeneration, optic nerve atrophy, retinal ischemia, macular degeneration, presbyopia, general poor eyesight...*How can I stop aging?*

Problem: Aging is a fact of life. It cannot be stopped. However, accelerated aging can be prevented by paying closer attention to lifestyle choices. All the tissues of the body are involved in the eyes; skin, nerve, muscle, connective tissue, blood, bone, lymph, and glands, all depend on a healthy immune system for optimum function. Due to its thinness, the periocular skin may show the earliest signs of aging, followed by connective tissue, muscles and organs, and later, nerve degeneration. Ophthalmologists have long been taught to consider the whole patient in our examination. Yet, we tend to focus our time on the eyes, and perhaps a little on the adjacent tissues. We ask patients about diabetes and hypertension and maybe a history of medications. We'll ask about trauma or previous surgeries and concentrate on the present complaints and symptoms. A family and social history may be elicited as pertaining to the chief complaint. Often ignored are the avoidable risk factors, such as the mental and emotional effects of stress, the unbalanced diet, poor elimination, toxin exposure, inadequate levels of physical activity, and other debilitating habits that lead to chronic inflammation and poor circulation.

Question: Why does one person age faster and more definitively than another? A large part of the answer may lie in lifestyle choices. Aging and bad habits reduce the function of body tissues more rapidly than aging alone. The choices one makes regarding nutrition, physical activity, social connections, and emotional attitude, plays a major role in determining the outcomes of old age. One may age gracefully with all senses intact, neurologically sound, physical fitness and mental alertness, or they may fall into an old-age scenario of immobility, physical suffering, and mental inertia.

To age without losing the basic functions (eyesight) and maintaining mobility should be a lifetime goal. This can be accomplished through making the right choices and living a healthy lifestyle.

A favorite truth and sometimes excuse for poor eyesight is genetics. "Well, my mother and father were blind, so I'm going to be blind too." Though genetics does play a significant role, the environment (and lifestyle choices) in which the genes must function, influences which genes are expressed and how much expression there will be. This expression determines the quality and quantity of life. Like hybrid vs. heritage (genotype) seeds, each has its own strengths and weaknesses, but it is the internal and external environment that shapes expression (phenotype). Genetics, like aging, is an unavoidable risk factor—altered gene expression, cell division errors, mutations, and dysfunctional DNA repair lead to loss of tissue function throughout the body, which accelerates aging. (1)

Mechanics of Aging/Causes of Aging: One of the principal mechanisms in the process of cellular aging involves telomere shortening as a result of use and time. Telomeres are the amino acids at the end of the chromosome that are normally lost with each cell division. The destruction and shortening of telomeres can be accelerated through poor lifestyle practices and prolonged body tissue abuse. Oxidative stress from both internal and external factors (toxicity from heavy metals, pollutants, poor nutrition, stresses, poor elimination, acute and chronic inflammation) leads to free radical damage, which adversely affects the aging process. Repression of the pineal gland reduces the release of melatonin, affecting rest patterns, and disrupting normal cell replication and repair. (2)

All parts of the eye are subject to accelerated aging. Abnormal accumulation of lipofucsin, amyloid and glycolated end-products leads to loss of membrane integrity and cell dysfunction. Dysfunction of lipid metabolism and dehydration of extracellular matrix are linked to arteriolarsclerosis, venous laxity, and poor circulation. Biochemical debris from metabolic processes accumulate in and between cells, disrupt cross links, glue cells to one another, cause mitochondrial failure, poison other cells, lead to mutations, adversely change extracellular matrix, and lead to physiologic decline. Studies indicate that these failures can be treated through repair rather than further blockage. (3) The effects of aging are due to multiple mechanisms and are accelerated under stress conditions. (4) (5) These stresses have a detrimental effect on the immune system and play an integral role accelerating the aging process and increased incidence of disease. A compromised immune system can lead to free proliferation of pathogens, unrestrained malignancies, endocrine dysfunction, allergic reactions, and uncontrolled inflammation resulting in progressive degeneration of cells, tissues, and organs.

Insult	Result	Solution
Oxidative Stress	free radical damage	antioxidants
Toxicity	heavy metals, pollutants (degenerative disease)	detoxification
Immune Dysfunction	impaired defense (inflammation)	adaptogens
Lipid Metabolism	poor cell function (cardiovascular collapse)	omega-3, B vitamins
Dehydration	poor circulation	cayenne, exercise
Weight Excess	obesity, body tissue stress	caloric restriction
Mental State	atrophy, disuse (impaired biorhythms)	attitude, social, spirituality, mental stimulation

Table 1. Basic Counteractive Treatment to Aging Processes:

Health: Good or bad health is not only related to genetics and environment, but is also a function of the way a person eats, drinks, feels, thinks, acts, and lives. Therefore a comprehensive health assessment plan for any individual will include diet and the nutrition derived from it, level of physical activity, mind-body emotional status, spiritual/social connections, internal energy, and external boosters or detractors. Since these factors affect the whole body, then eye tissues are adversely affected by poor quality nutrition, poor elimination (accumulation of toxins), proinflammation habits, inadequate rest, lack of exercise (poor circulation), and dysfunctional immune system.

"A healthy body and an active mind have everything to do with healthy eyes."

—A.L. Anduze

Vitamin C	Vitamin E	Lutein	Zinc
citrus fruit	soy	spinach	legumes
melons	greens	kale	dried beans
tomatoes	fish	collards	garbanzo beans
potatoes	wheat germ	romaine	chickpeas
broccoli	nuts	peas	black-eyed peas
	seeds	berries	soy

Table 2. Antioxidants for Aging

Patient Education: The doctor provides information to the patient about eye diseases in the form of brochures, newsletters, and digital media. Modern eye care should include a distinct section on *patient responsibility* and attitude. A negative attitude impairs health. A positive attitude enhances health. Depressed feelings and negative speech regarding the inability to perform optimally or poor outcomes need to be addressed from a realistic point of view. Too often only the doctor is held responsible. Patients need to take responsibility for their own health status, actions and behavior. How one ages, greatly influences treatment outcomes.

"There are 120 medical schools to teach one how to become a doctor and not one school to teach one how to behave as a patient."

—Anonymous

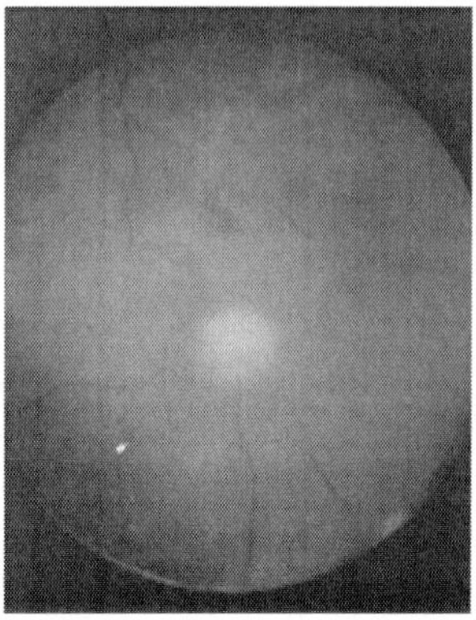

atrophic nerve & retina in a 92 year old

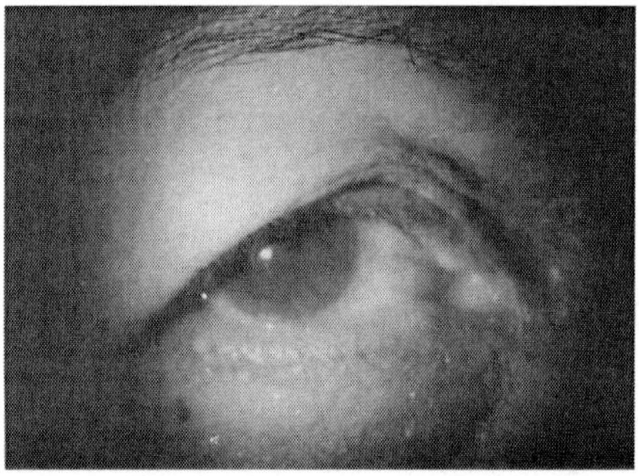

dermatochalasis in a 75 year old

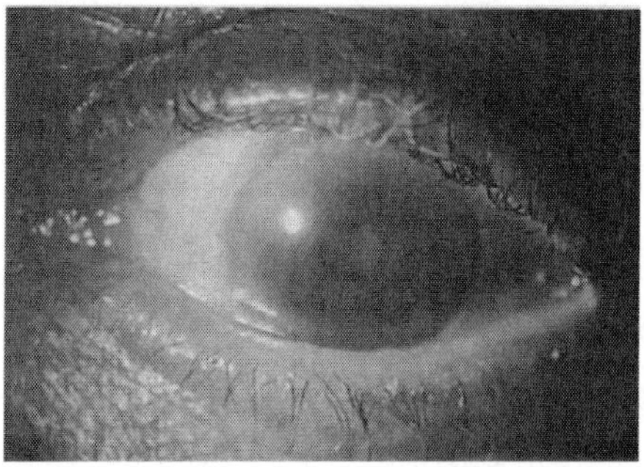

arcus senilis and brunescent cataract in an 80 year old

Aging Strategies/Solutions: Cellular DNA undergoes continuous damage (oxidation) and subsequent repair. (6) Basic therapeutic and behavioral strategies exist, which can favorably influence the repair process and perhaps delay the decline of body tissue. By far, the most effective evidence-based strategy for preserving neural cells is through regular and repetitive aerobic physical activity. Exercise improves the efficiency of blood perfusion, counters depression through hormonal regulation (endorphins), improves bone-muscle strength, and helps regulate blood glucose. Good nutrition directed at the reduction of inflammation improves both the immune system and effective DNA repair mechanisms.

Obesity hastens the aging process. Through weight control, the principles of extreme caloric-restricting diets to promote longevity can be applied to eye tissues. People with higher than normal abdominal adiposity have lower telomere lengths. (7) Eating less, but with more nutrients, and eating more often is crucial to body tissue maintenance: Reducing toxicity through better hydration, proper elimination, detoxification practices, and avoidance is an integral part of regulating the aging process. Avoiding nutritional overload and insulin resistance will help to avoid type 2 diabetes, which is a major cause of eye pathology. Consuming less protein, more fiber, good fats, and antioxidants will promote cellular repair. Reduce unnecessary stress; the release of the stress hormone, cortisol, can lead to weight gain and shrink the hippocampus, the center of thought and memory vital to regulation of the aging process.

Case Scenario Two:A 56-year-old patient with dry eyes due to a combination of dehydration and ocular surface dysfunction, presents with oily tear film and scattered lid margin flakes, which is due to a meibomian gland dysfunction. She has a history of chronic allergies, treated with multiple topical and systemic antihistaminics.

Conventional treatments include a trial on artificial tears (three types), followed by medications (cyclosporine to increase goblet cells) should work, but sometimes do not. Loteprednol, administered to reduce inflammatory factors also offers no relief. Aqueous deficiency may be a significant factor as punctum plugs may give some relief.

Complimentary Treatment of Dry Eyes:

1. Avoidance of excess alcohol (a drying agent), as well as excess sun and exposure to chemical or physical irritants.
2. Hydration (drink six to eight glasses of water per day regularly).
3. Omega-3 (flaxseed oil). (8) (9)

These adjunctive therapies are logical and easy and involve simple dialogue and common sense.

Environmental Geriatrics: Where and how an individual lives can certainly affect his/her health. Aging rates are often related to economic status and location in that one's access to health care in the form of health education, early diagnosis, effective treatment, and in the United States, ability to pay for such care can be beneficial or detrimental. In addition, a good supportive environment with adequate safety features can make a difference between function and dysfunction.

Economics and politics are beyond the scope of this book, but patients with low vision can benefit from a number of simple, inexpensive adjustments in their homes.

Task List of Situational Improvements:

1. Windows and doors should be easy to open and close.
2. *Good lighting* especially in the bathroom and kitchen. Not all people with low vision need stronger lights than those with normal vision. People with macular degeneration and

glaucoma may require higher light levels, whereas those with central (cortical or subcapsular) cataracts may prefer lower light levels. Lighting levels should be adjusted on an individual basis. Glare—poor vision as a result of direct or reflected light—may result from incorrect bulbs or the presence of overly reflective surfaces. Use a flexible neck floor lamp instead of a table lamp for reading. Try chromalux or full-spectrum incandescent bulb 75–100 watts for close-up task lighting and 150–300 watts incandescent or fluorescent bulbs for room lighting. A 60-watt bulb placed 12–16 inches from the task is good for optimal function. Frosted or soft white bulbs are easier on the eyes. Be aware of the heat generated by incandescent bulbs when on for a long period of time. On the other hand, a cool white light with a bluish tinge (full-spectrum fluorescent) may be more comfortable for people with low vision. A 3-way bulb with a dimmer switch can control the amount of lighting in a room. Light all stairs well with switches that can be turned on and off from upstairs or down. Make sure that all outdoor walkways, paths, and the entrance foyer are well lit.

3. Use *contrasting colors* in and around the home to emphasize light switch plates, outlets, doorsills, edges of coffee tables and bathtubs. Planting brightly colored flowers along walkways, and using white or brightly colored plates on dark tables or vice versa, can greatly enhance the ability of an individual with low vision to see important objects and areas.
4. Use a variety of *textures*, like Velcro, rubber bands, and raised dots to identify edges, objects, or controls within the home. Choose matte finish for floors and furniture and cover windows with blinds and drapes to reduce glare.

5. Make *black print* on white background labels to identify on/off switches, appliances, and potential hazards, and ask the pharmacist for large print on medicine bottles.
6. Avoid tripping hazards such as loose rugs, irregular floors, tub and shower access, and stairs.
7. Make a resource list of companies and outlets in your area that provide low vision aids and guides and use them.(10)

Exercise	regular, 30 minutes, 3 times a week
Nutrition	weight control, antioxidants, multivitamin, immune system boosters, reduce inflammation, proper digestion and elimination, detoxification, hydration
Stress Factors	breathing techniques, B vitamins, adaptogens, color and sound therapy
Mental State	stimulation for increased brain circulation, adequate rest
Avoid Risky Behavior	toxins, dehydration, poor diet, infectious pathogens, inflammatory stimuli

Table 3. Recommendations of Lifestyle Strategies for Healthy Aging

> "Lifestyle interventions made at age 45 with benefit the individual at age 90."
>
> —A.L.Anduze

References for Chapter One:

1. Ly DH, Lockhart DJ, Lerner RA, Schultz PG. Mitotic Misregulation and Human Aging. Science. 2000 Mar 31; 287(5462):2486–92
2. Andrew Weil, MD. Healthy Aging: why we age. Anchor Books 2005, p.82–103
3. Phoenix C, de Grey AD. A model of aging as accumulated damage matches observed mortality patterns and predicts the life-extending effects of prospective interventions. Age (Dordr.) 2007 Dec 29 (4):133–89
4. Rubin H. Cell aging in vivo and in vitro. Mech Ageing Dev. 1997 Oct; 98(1):1–35
5. Jazwinski SM. Longevity, genes, and aging. Science. 1996 Jul 5; 273(5271):54–9

6. Friedberg EC. DNA damage and repair. Nature. 2003 Jan 23; 421(6921):436–40
7. Lee M, etal. Inverse association between adiposity and telomere length: The fels longitudinal study. Am J Hum Biol. 2010 Nov 15.
8. Wojtowicz JC, etal. Pilot, Prospective, Randomized, Double-masked, Placebo-controlled Clinical Trial of an Omega-3 Supplement for Dry Eye. Cornea. 2010 Oct 28.
9. Pinheiro MN Jr. etal. Oral flaxseed oil (Linum usitatissimum) in the treatment for dry-eye Sjögren's syndrome patients. Arg Bras Oftalmol. 2007 Jul–Aug; 70(4):649–55.
10. Bakker, R. Household Tips for People with Low Vision. www.cornellEG.org

Inflammation and Immunity

Of the high-risk factors for eye disease, the following conditions are more susceptible to inflammation and therefore commonly lead to damage at the cellular level: Systemic hypertension (with arterial damage), high cholesterol and triglycerides (arteriolosclerosis), diabetes mellitus (high blood glucose levels), and obesity (high adipokines, free fatty acids, and lipoproteins).

(WHO report 2002: Global Strategy on Diet, Physical Activity and Health) (1)

Case Scenario One: Five cataract surgeries have been scheduled, four of which present with clinical evidence of arthritis, hypertension, type 2 diabetes, as well as other age-related debilitations. Additionally, two patients have C-reactive protein levels >5.0 and none of the patients' eyes show flare and cells on slit lamp exam. Visual acuities are less than 20/200 in all five. How can these cases be managed by the ophthalmologist?

Three cases could be approached with medium risk. The remaining two patient cases should be postponed, pending the reduction of inflammation levels via dietary changes and improvements and oral medications over a four- to six-week period. These two patients are considered higher risk for postoperative inflammatory complications, especially vascular. Once the CRP levels are stabilized at 3.0 or less and the other lab values reflect results closer to normal, a better surgical outcome is expected should the physician elect to proceed.

C-reactive protein is a highly sensitive marker for inflammation, particularly in arteries, and is linked to thrombosis in veins. In chronic uncontrolled diabetes, high glucose, adipokines, free fatty acids, and lipoproteins stimulate CRP production in arterial endothelial cells, which in turn leading to increased inflammation and vascular pathology. (2) CRP is a good predictor of cardiovascular disease. (3) High CRP levels are associated with risk of age-related macular disease (Rotterdam Study). Smoking, high alcohol intake, high body mass index, and diets consisting of a high glycemic index each raise CRP levels; low-to-moderate alcohol intake, diets consisting of low glycemic index, statins, and multivitamins all reduce CRP levels. (4) (5) (6)

Surgery is traumatic and if the inflammation response for normal wound healing is compromised or enhanced by systemic disorders, there is a higher risk for complicated outcomes. It is well accepted that patients with ocular surface disease, uveitis, and diabetic retinopathy require more attention preoperatively, intraoperatively and postoperatively than those patients without. Patients with high CRP levels and atherosclerosis, arthritis, diabetes, hypertension, acute infection, and autoimmune disorders also require more attention preoperatively.

> "Most eye diseases involve some form of immune system dysfunction and inflammation."
>
> —Consensus of Ophthalmologists

Brief Summary of the Inflammatory Response:

1. (Trauma/Antigenic Insult) -> stimulation of preformed mediators
2. Early release of cytokines (reduced by corticosteroids, Cox-1 inhibitors) -> prostaglandin E2 and leukotriene C4, histamines, bradykinins, SRS (slow-reacting substance) from mast cells and platelet-activating factor, interleukin-1, and others initiate an instant attack on

target tissues (e.g. ocular surface diseases, blepharitis, conjunctivitis, allergic, viral, and bacterial)
3. (Persistence of insult) -> release of cytokines IL-1 and TNF
4. Activation of the endothelial cells to up-regulate VCAM-1, ICAM-1, E-selectin, L-selectin
5. Increases neutrophils, monocytes, activated T-helper, T-cytotoxic, memory T and B cells, (e.g. uveitis, graft rejection, vasculitis)
6. Late release of Cox-2 enzymes (reduced by aspirin and NSAIDs) -> inflammation hormones (arachidoninc acid (omega-6 fatty acids) in cell membranes and walls), and newly formed inflammatory mediators are produced through activation of phospholipase A
7. Recruitment of inflammatory cells (WBCs) -> increased production of more mediators
8. Tissue destruction -> *organ dysfunction*(7)

Recommendations to reduce inflammation preoperatively and boost immunity postoperatively.

1. In addition to the preoperative reduction of inflammation with topical and systemic steroids restore the immune system to a normal or near-normal status for handling the inflammatory response to surgery. Use a phosphate base topical steroid (dexamethasone 0.1 percent) as it tends not to cross the cornea as readily as an acetate, and/or cyclosporine or loteprednol drops qid.
2. Do not continue steroids indefinitely (as in arthritis and uveitis) as they suppress the healing process.
3. Do CRP levels, and/or vitamin and mineral levels and antioxidant levels if available to measure and monitor the inflammation status.

4. Initiate an anti-inflammation diet-a with reduction in omega-6 foods and increase foods that reduce inflammation. (Table 1)
5. Use *cold* preservative-free tears at least qid and a mild decongestant with.012 percent Naphazoline bid as indicated.
6. Operate on a *quiet eye* and do minimal damage to tissues.
7. Boost the immune system with diet-b of immune enhancing foods (Table 2) and vitamin C 300–500 mg and zinc 25 mg bid, omega-3 1000 mg, garlic (one clove), ginger 500 mg, turmeric 800 mg for two weeks preoperatively, if possible.
8. Avoid overuse of steroids and antibiotics postoperatively in non-implant cases.

During the immediate postoperative period, promotion of wound healing should be preferred over immune suppression, especially in cases not involving implants. The prevention and control of inflammation is the key to a successful outcome. With a sound immune system, healing will occur without the disruption of an excessive inflammatory response.

Avoid or reduce intake of pro inflammatory omega-6 products.

Fried foods	Packaged foods	White sugar	Red meat
Processed wheat (gluten)	Polyunsaturated vegetable oils	Monosodium glutamate (MSG)	High fructose corn syrup (HFCS)
Caffeine	Excess alcohol	Peanuts	Dairy products

Table 1. Anti-inflammation Diet-A

Avoid or reduce intake: Proinflammatory omega-6 products (corn, safflower oil, partially hydrogenated vegetable oils, cooking oil that *smokes*, mayonnaise, salad dressings, white flour, white rice, instant mashed potatoes, egg yolks, poultry skin, more than two *drinks* a day)

Increase intake of omega-3 products, antioxidants, low protein whole foods

Vegetables	Fruits (berries)	Beans & legumes	Pasta	Whole grains
Extra virgin olive oil, flaxseed oil	Walnuts and seeds	Mushrooms (cooked)	Fish/seafood (wild)	whole soy plant based foods
Mushrooms	Lean meats	Garlic	Ginger & turmeric	Cinnamon
Avocados	Dark chocolate	Red wine *	Yogurt	Green tea

Table 2. Anti-inflammation Diet-B

Increase intake: Omega-3 products, antioxidants, low-protein whole foods

*Cocoa-enriched diets enhance expression of phosphatases and decrease inflammatory molecules. (8)

*Resveratrol in red wine blocks the production of inflammation triggers, sphingosine kinase and phospholipase D. (9)

Bioflavonoids (proanthocyanisins) in fruits and vegetables have antioxidant, antitumor, anti-inflammation, and antiallergic activity.

Adequate water intake is essential for proper cellular function.

Case Scenario Two: A 34-year-old female presents with bilateral red eyes, tearing, swollen caruncles, and a thin mucus discharge. She imparts a history of allergies for which she uses topical over-the-counter antihistamines and oral tablets from her family doctor. She admits to vigorous eye rubbing on a daily basis. She asks, "Why are my eyes so red, and what else can I do besides using eyedrops?"

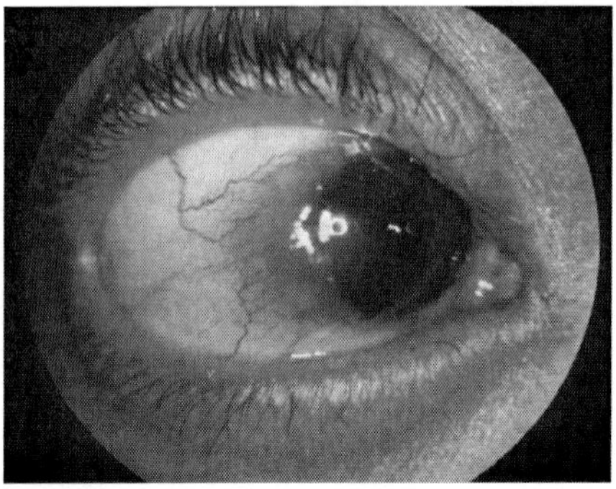

vernal keratoconjunctivitis/ limbal catarrh

Type 1 hypersensitivity, an allergic reaction, results from an inappropriate immune response that triggers acute inflammation. In response to allergens, conjunctival mast cells release vasoactive chemicals, including histamines, leukotrienes, and basophils (chemotaxis and swelling); this is later followed by the release of cytokines, eosinophils, and other proinflammatory molecules, which propagate an excessive inflammatory response with characteristics of hyperemia, epiphora, and severe itching (See Figure 1). (10) The repetition of such episodes may lead to tissue damage and lesions, as in Figure 2. Topical and systemic antihistamines inhibit the symptoms only temporarily and they often return with a rebound.

Recommendations for Red Eyes Due to Allergies:

1. Conventional therapy for acute symptoms.
2. Rest: Improve digestion and elimination.
3. Increase water intake: Flush tissues and keep mucus surfaces moist.
4. Increase omega-3, antioxidant-rich fruits (berries) to reduce the inflammation response.
5. Stinging nettle extract (Urtica dioica) (fried-dried capsules 300 mg) with antioxidant, diuretic, and anti-inflammatory effects; blocks both COX-1 and COX-2 inhibitors; and

butterbur (Petasites hybridus) (extract tablets): Both are good as antihistamines but without the drowsiness. (11) (12) (Butterbur should only be used short term due to reported side effects of liver toxicity and cancer)

6. Acupuncture. (13)

Ginger (*Zingiber off.*) 300-500mg	Turmeric (*Curcuma longa) 600*-800 mg	*Boswellia serrata* 400-1200 mg
Cats claw (250-1000mg)	Bromelain (A*nanas com.*)	Devils claw (600-1200mg),
Guggul (500-1000mg)	Cayenne (C*apsaicin*)	Fenugreek
Echinacea purpura	Eyebright (*Euphrasia off.)*	*Argemone mexicana*

Table 3. Botanicals for Inflammation:

These botanicals are mainly COX-2 inhibitors, which suppress the synthesis of prostaglandins like NSAIDs but without the side effects. They are taken orally.

Ginger inhibits or deactivates genes in the body that encode molecules of chronic inflammation.

Turmeric prevents production of prostaglandins and deactivates inflammation-regulating genes through the effects of gene signaling.

Cayenne pepper is an antioxidant that reduces the pain of inflammation.

Echinacea root has known antimicrobial, antiviral, and anti-inflammatory properties. (See Immune enhancers)

Eyebright leaves should be cut, sun-dried, steeped in a cup of boiled water for seven to ten minutes, strained, poured into a dropper bottle and refrigerated for twenty-four hours. Use one drop to eyes three to four times daily until symptoms disappear. It may also be taken as an infusion for general inflammation reduction. (14), (15 (16) (17)

Case Scenario Three: A 56-year-old female presents with mild conjunctival congestion. She reports that her eyes are always dry and gritty. She has tried all the drops and gadgets and does not wish to have any surgery. She asks, "What else can I do to get some relief?"

Dry eyes are often associated with blepharitis, conjunctivitis, keratitis, chronic use of topical medications preservatives, contact lenses, and increased pathogens on the ocular surface. Besides anatomic or chemical denervation, the causes are usually associated with decreased levels of aqueous, oil and /or mucus in the composition of the tear film.

Recommendations for Dry Eyes:

1. In addition to conventional treatments with topical tear film lubricants, cyclosporine, corticosteroids, punctal plugs, oral doxycycline, autologous serum drops, acetylcysteine, moisture goggles.
2. Increase basic hydration (six to eight glasses of water daily) and one extra for each juice or beverage imbibed.Drink juices diluted. Reduce or discontinue alcohol intake.
3. Look for and control allergies; note that most antihistamines are dehydrating agents.
4. Omega-3 fish oil (450mg EPA, 300mg DHA) and/or 1000mg Flaxseed oil) taken daily (showed significant increase in average tear production and volume) (*18*) (*19*)

Recommendations for Prevention of Eye Infections:

1. Never touch your eyes with your hands (unless washed).
2. Change towels, face cloths, and pillowcases often.
3. Avoid contaminated eye make-up or mascara.
4. Do not share eye make-up, washcloth, or towel with others.
5. Do not touch eyedrop bottle to eye.
6. Keep infected children out of school until clears.

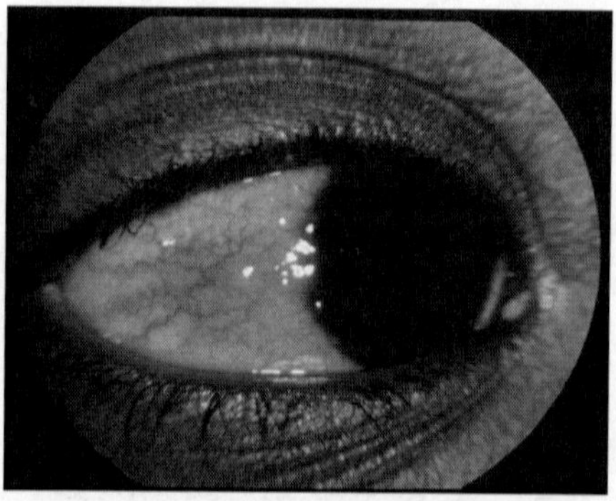

inflamed & infected eye

Recommendations for Red Eyes From Infection and Inflammatory Lesions:

1. Conventional treatment with antibiotics for bacteria, not viruses or allergies, and immune suppressants (corticosteroids) for acute inflammation.
2. Treat dry eyes with topical tear film lubricants and general hydration.
3. Anti-inflammation diet-a and -b.
4. *Calendula officinalis* (marigold) tincture used topically bid has significant antibacterial activity. (20)

Recommendations for Natural Anti-Inflammatory Measures:

1. Exercise decreases stress hormones and inflammation mediators in the blood stream.
2. Rest helps recuperation and body healing.
3. Discontinue bad habits like smoking, excess alcohol intake, caffeine, and stimulant drugs.

4. Go *green* with cleaner surroundings. Replace air fresheners with natural houseplants like rhododendrons, English ivy (*Hedera helix*), ferns (*Asparagus densiflorus*), waxy leafed plants (*Hoya carnosa*), purple heart (*Tradescantia pallida*) or purple waffle (*Hemigraphus alternate*). To fix a *sick building*, call OSHA 1-800-321-6742 or go to www.osha.gov for more information.
5. Reduce exposure to environmental toxins and consider a gentle detoxification two to three times a year.
6. Consider alternative pain management in place of strong toxic pain medications.

Case Scenario Four: "My eye got red, just like that! It doesn't hurt, but it looks awful. I didn't get hit and I don't have any blood pressure problems or other medical conditions that I know of."

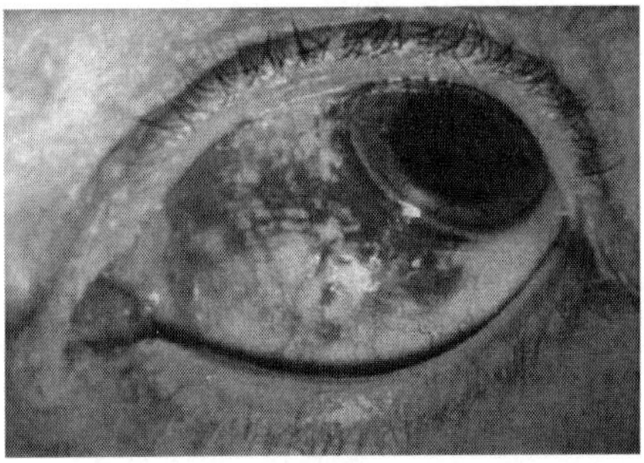

subconjunctival hemorrhage

Recommendations for spontaneous conjunctival hemorrhage:

1. In addition to conventional treatments to prevent bacterial proliferation and further bleeding.
2. Get history of use of botanicals and supplements, which may inhibit platelet activity and prolong blood coagulation: Garlic, *Ginkgo biloba*, ginger, ginseng root, goldenseal, devil's claw, echinacea, feverfew, fish oil, grapefruit juice, flaxseed, danshen, dong quai, cayenne, turkey tail,

licorice, coenzyme Q10, glucosamine-chondroitin, all have coumarin-like effects. Educate and discontinue use until healed.
3. Discontinue aspirin, NSAIDs, and Plavix use.
4. Apply cold compress or eyewash for the vasoconstrictive effects.

Inflammation of the deeper layers of the eye (uvea, sclera, vitreous, retina, and choroid) represents a spectrum of ocular disorders that involve contiguous structures. The diagnosis of specific syndromes is usually made through a combination of pattern recognition, associated with systemic signs and symptoms and laboratory and imaging studies. The routine use of a broad panel of studies is discouraged as many are nonspecific. The mainstay of treatment remains corticosteroids due to their rapid onset and multiple effects on inflammation. Long-term use is limited due to a variety of local and systemic side effects. The use of NSAIDs, though somewhat reduced in efficacy, is recommended in its stead, but long-term side effects such as hepatotoxicity, hypothalamic-pituitary-adrenal axis impairment, metabolic acidosis, and cost have also been noted. (21) (22)

Most severe or chronic diseases have an element of immune dysfunction at the central core of the process. Many age-related degenerative diseases like Alzheimer's, multiple sclerosis, and macular degeneration are linked to autoimmune inflammatory responses. There is an inverse risk relationship between AD and use of NSAIDS. (23) Nutritional deficiencies are also significantly involved in the maintenance of immunity and inflammation and linked to diabetes and uveitis and possibly glaucoma. Vitamin D deficiency affects the mechanisms of immune cells and increases the risk of infections and inflammatory diseases. Vitamin A is a key modulator of TGF beta, which suppresses cytokines. Vitamin E deficiency is associated with overproduction of immature T cells and unchecked prostaglandin generation. (24)

A compromised immune system can lead to the manifestation of infections, allergies, malignancies, endocrine dysfunction, inflammation, and chronic inflammatory systemic diseases. Inflammation influences the environment around tumor cells, contributing to proliferation, migration, and survival. Cancer cells use selectins, chemokines, and their receptors as vehicles for invasion of tissues and to enable metastasis; likewise, some inflammatory cells contribute to cancer inhibition. (35)

Recommendations for Complimentary Treatment of Autoimmune, Autoinflammatory, and Neoplastic diseases:

1. Discontinue all bad habits. Many autoimmuine and inflammatory diseases are associated with environmental and ingested toxins (exposure to free radicals).
2. Reduce stress levels. Increased serum cortisol has been associated with electrolyte imbalance and infection. (25)

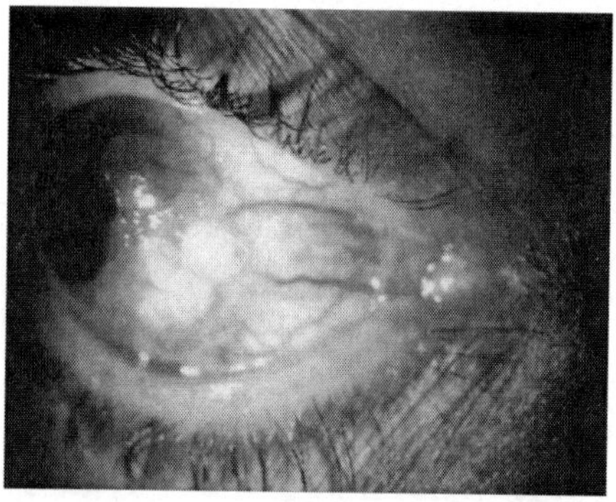

squamous cell carcinoma

3. In addition to conventional medical treatment and with the approval of the treating physician, be careful about using steroid suppression and immune boosters at same time. In certain cases it may be counterproductive. It may be practical to reduce the acute inflammation first with suppression, then boost immune system with enhancers.

4. The anti-inflammation diet should be a mainstay. (Adapted from the books of Andrew Weil, MD)
5. Medical mushrooms (reischii, maitake, shiitake) against cancer, allergies and infections build strong white blood cells.
6. Anticancer foods. (See Table 4)
7. Reduce inflammatory markers like C-reactive protein and homocysteine.
8. Multivitamins and minerals: Vitamin A (betacarotenoids) increase white blood cells; C blocks free radical damage and increases white blood cells; E increases killer T cells; B6 (pyridoxine) increases lymphocyte proliferation and interleukin production; B12 (cobalamin) increases protein and red blood cell production and nerve cell membrane integrity; and zinc increases white blood cells and T cells.
9. Goji berries enhance the antioxidant activity of vitamins A, C, and E.
10. Eleutherocides increase T lymphocytes and ginsenocides reduce the stress hormone, cortisol, and increase the production of T-helper cells.
11. *Tylophora indica* (200–400 mg) anti-inflammatory and antihistaminic for arthritis, bronchitis, and asthma.

Green tea (*Camellia sinensis*)	Lemongrass (*Cymbopogon flex.*.)	Astragalus root (*A.membranaceus*)	Leafy greens
Garlic (*Allium sativum)*	Almonds, Amaranth, Apples, Broccoli	Barley, Beans, Beets, Bok choy	Brussels sprouts
Carrots	Celery	Cereal grasses	Chickpeas, Corn
Figs	Ginger	Horseradish	Lentils, Mllet
Canola &Olive oil	Onion	Parsley	Potatoes
Purslane	Radishes	Mints	Turmeric

Table 4. Anticancer Foods and Botanicals

Green tea has polyphenolic compounds (epigallocatechins), which impart protection against cancer through increased formation and excretion of metabolites of carcinogens. (26)

Lemongrass has citrals, which make cancer cells destroy themselves through apoptosis. (27)

Astragalus root stimulates white blood cell production and inhibits chemo-induced immunosuppression. (28)

Leafy greens contain antioxidant folates which protect against free radicals.

Garlic has the antioxidant selenium and organic sulfur compounds, which promote early mitotic arrest followed by apoptotic cell death without affecting healthy cells. (29)

Almonds, amaranth, barley, broccoli, beets, bok choy, chickpeas, corn, lentils, millet, and potatoes have a variety of protease inhibitors (antibiotics, alkaloids, terpenes, lectins, etc.) which block cancer cell initiation and contribute to the plants' defense against pests and pathogens.

Carrots, celery, cereal grasses, ginger, turmeric, radishes, and purslane are rich in antioxidants and carotenoids.

Figs (*Ficus carica*) have the anticancer phytochemical, benzaldehyde, which exhibits very high antitumor activity. (30)

Recommendations for Strengthening the Immune System through Complimentary Therapies:

1. Encounter and endure less stress. The adrenal glands produce epinephrine, norepinephrine, and cortisol. Acute stress boosts the immune system while chronic stress wears it out. Psychological stress aggravates allergies, asthma, inflammatory and autoimmune diseases. In many cases, massage therapy, spa treatments, meditation, music, and the arts can relieve stress. (31)
2. Moderate exercise can stimulate the redistribution of leukocytes in the blood. (32)

3. Sleeping soundly can stimulate growth hormones, the repair of DNA and the immune system, and it can also decrease the production of inflammatory chemicals. (33)
4. Social connections are good for healthy body systems.
5. Avoid toxins (tobacco, excess alcohol, air pollutants) (Chapter 3: The Toxic Eye)
6. Consume live friendly bacteria. (Yogurt, sauerkraut, kimchi...*probiotics*)
7. Choose vitamins and supplements wisely. Avoid deficiencies of vitamin C, A, E, B6, selenium, zinc, and folic acid. Be aware that excess vitamin A can be toxic and too much zinc can cause immune system dysfunction (anemia, leucopenia, neutropenia).(34)

Echinacea *(E. purpura)*	Garlic (*Allium sativa)*	Turmeric (*Curcuma longa*)	Reischi mushroom (*Ganoderma luc.*)
Shiitake mushroom (*Lentinus edodes*)	Green tea (*Camillia sinensis)*	Goldenseal(*Hydrasti s canadensis)*	Ginger (*Zingiber off.)*
Panax ginseng	Omega 3 FFA	Cinnamon	Astragalus
Cat's claw	Grapeseeds	Vitamin C	Kelp
Probiotics			

Table 5. Immune System Enhancers:

Echinacea reversed the acute inflammation response in acne and brings cytokine levels back to normal, (36) but had no significant effect on the common cold when compared to a placebo in one study. (37)

Garlic counteracts glutathione loss during the inflammation process and curtails the activities of catalase and superoxide dismutase enzymes. (38) Thiacremonone, a sulfur compound from garlic extract, exerts its anti-inflammatory activity through the inhibition of NF-kB. (39)

Turmeric, reischi, and shiitake mushrooms enhance innate immunity by increasing the levels of mRNA in macrophages. (40) The epigallocatechins in green tea inhibit adhesion and migration of B cells in the blood by blocking CD11b and the polysaccharides enhance the phagocytic activity of macrophage-like cells. (41) (42) Goldenseal treatment shows an increase in the primary IgM response to antigenic stimulation. (43)

Ginger acts to restore an impaired humoral immune response. (44)

Panax ginseng triggers immune responses through prevention of macrophage cell regression caused by antigenic activity.

Omega-3 free fatty acids (EPA, DHA, GLA) improve macrophage function in cases of defective phagocytosis of apoptotic cells. (46)

Cinnamon polyphenol extract (CPE) can affect immune responses by regulating anti- and proinflammatory and GLUT gene expression. (47)

Astragalus polysaccharides can regulate T cell-mediated immunity via CD11c (high) CD45RB (low)

DCs in vitro. (48)

Cat's claw (and echinacea) may modulate the immune system through activation of macrophages. (49)

The proanthocyanin from grape seeds potentiates antitumor activity of doxorubicin (DOX). (50)

Vitamin C down-regulates VEGF production via the modulation of COX-2 expression. (51)

The sodium alginate in kelp can enhance innate immunity and disease resistance against invasive bacteria. (52)

A probiotics-enriched diet can restore the altered haemotological parameters and enhance innate immunity in some bacterial infections. (53)

Pro Cancerous Foods, Additives and Habits:

1. Partially dehydrogenated vegetable oils
2. Alfalfa sprouts have L-canavanine which worsens autoimmunity.
3. Foods with sodium nitrite, hydrogenated oils, & refined carbohydrates

4. Sodium nitrate in packaged meat products
5. Aspartame, saccharin and artificial colorings
6. Cigarette smoking
7. Excessive sunblock or sunlight
8. Avoiding physical exercise
9. Poor general nutrition (insufficient carbohydrates, good fats, protein)
10. Excessive radiation and chemotherapy

All of these play a role in compromising and/or destroying the immune system.

Case Scenario Five: A 45-year-old male sustains a laceration to his left eyebrow and lid in a motor vehicle accident. He is seriously concerned about eyelid dysfunction and possible scar tissue disfigurement after the repair and asks what else he can do to help the wound healing process.

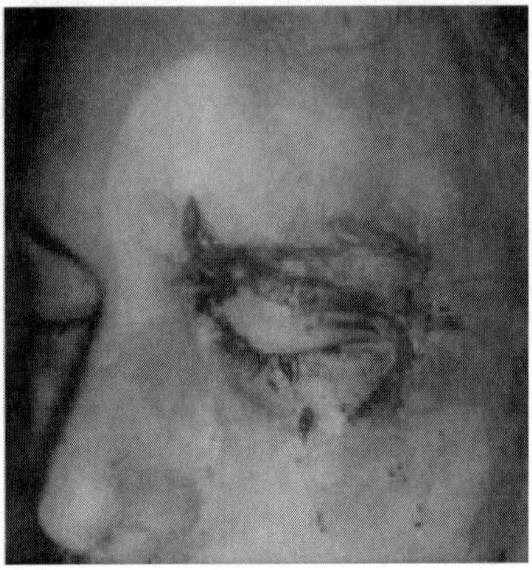

brow & lid laceration

Wound healing occurs in four basic steps: Initial hemostasis, reactive inflammation, cell proliferation, and collagen remodeling. Any agents that enhance or protect these phases greatly assist the healing process. He was instructed that there are several foods and supplements that contain vitamins and minerals which assist with wound healing. After primary laceration suture repair, the patient chose to take a multivitamin, omega-3 capsules, and *Aloe vera* drops. The aloe drops were prepared from fresh plants located within our laboratory facility. Though it was not a completely sterile preparation and not enhanced (or diluted) with preservatives, there were no adverse effects to its use. We were all pleased with the results.

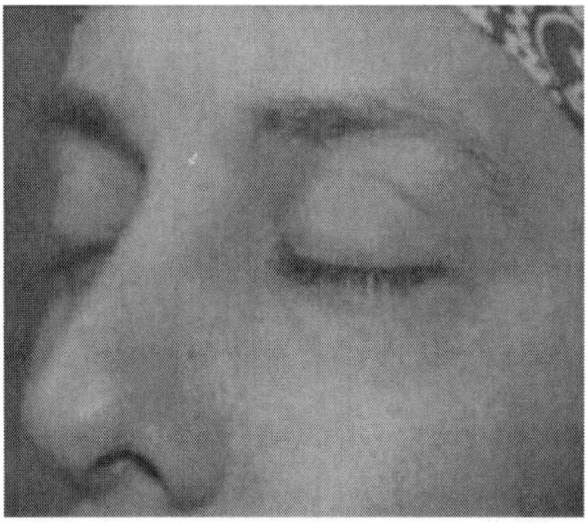

good healing & complete function after 10 weeks

Recommendations for healthy wound healing:

1. Vitamin C 500–1000 mg.
2. Zinc 25 mg.
3. Vitamin A 10,000 IU.
4. Vitamin E 400 IU.
5. Omega-3 fish oil 1000 mg.
6. Garlic (one clove).
7. *Aloe vera* drops tid.
8. Bitter melon (*Mormordica charantia*) extract tid.

All or any combination may be used.
(54) (55) (56) (57) (58) (59) (60)

Aloe vera, most commonly found in dry tropical areas, is the medicinal plant known as the *plant doctor*. Of the 240-specie variations, four are significant: A. arborescens, A. barbadensis, A. Vera, and A. vulgaris. The outer leaf encloses a free-flowing liquid, which acts as a laxative for internal use. The inner gel contains the moisturizing and wound-healing ingredients, anthroquinones (aloe-emodin, aloin, and barbaloin), polysaccharides (glucomannan, acemannan, and bradykininase), carboxypeptidase, magnesium lactate, zinc, calcium, glucose, cholesterol, salicylic acid, saponins, lignins, plant sterols, amino acids, prostaglandin precursors, antioxidants, and a generous supply of vitamins C, E, and A. These constituents stimulate fibroblasts to make collagen, activate macrophages, increase blood flow, and produce cytokines and other cell mediators, which appear to accelerate the healing process.

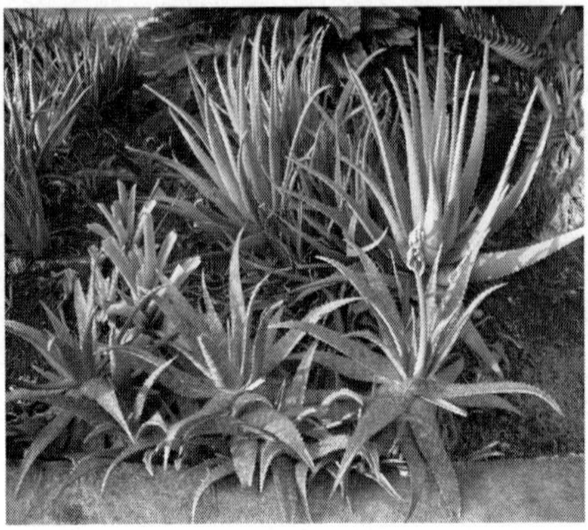

aloe vera & aloe vulgaris in the garden

Recommendation for *Aloe vera* drop preparation for closed external wounds:

1. Cut one frond and remove three teaspoons of gel.

2. Put into a shallow glass dish and add boiled water to 50 percent dilution.
3. Macerate and mix until dissolved.
4. Transfer to an amber or dark bottle (2 oz) and shake thoroughly.
5. Place in the refrigerator for twenty-four hours.
6. Use tid or qid to affected area for six to twelve weeks.

Side effects include the possibility of skin irritation in hypersensitive individuals.

The solution changes color after three to four days and should be discarded and a new solution made.

(The role of inflammation in age-related macular disease risk will be presented and discussed in Chapter 4.)

References for Chapter Two:

1. World Health Organization: Global Strategy on Diet, Physical Activity and Health. Chronic disease risk factors: WHO Report 2002.
2. Mugabo Y, Li L, Renier G. The connection between C-reactive protein (CRP) and diabetic vasculopathy. Focus on preclinical findings. Curr Diabetes Rev. 2010 Jan; 6(1):27-34.
3. Pfützner A et al. High –sensitivity C-reactive protein predicts cardiovascular risk in diabetic and nondiabetic patients: effects of insulin-sensitizing treatment with pioglitazone.J Diabetes Sci Technol. 2010 May 1; 4(3):706-16.
4. Blum S et al. Effect of a Mediterranean meal on postprandial carotenoids, paraoxonase activity and C-reactive protein levels. Ann Nutr Metab. 2006; 50(1):20-4.
5. Boekhoorn SS et al. C-reactive protein level and risk of aging macula disorder: The Rotterdam Study. Arch Ophthalmol. 2007 Oct; 125 (10):1396-401.
6. The Heart Protection Study Group: Collaborative Group C-reactive protein concentration and the vascular benefits of statin

therapy: an analysis of 20 536 patients in the Heart Protection Study. The Lancet, 28 January 2011,

7. Feghali CA, Wright TM. Cytokines in acute and chronic inflammation. Front Biosci. 1997 Jan 1; d12-26.
8. Cady RJ, Durham PL. Cocoa-enriched diets enhance expression of phosphatases and decrease expression of inflammatory molecules in trigeminal ganglion neurons. Brain Res.2010 Apr 6; 1323:18-32.
9. Issuree PD et al.Resveratrol attenuates C5a-induced inflammatory responses in vitro and in vivo by inhibiting phospholipase D and sphingosine kinase activities. FASEB J. 2009 Aug; 23(8):2412-24.
10. Cook EB.Tear cytokines in acute and chronic ocular allergic inflammation. Curr Opin Allergy Clin Immunol. 2004 Oct; 4(5):441-5.
11. Roschek B Jr et al. Nettle extract (Urtica dioica) affects key receptors and enzymes associated with allergic rhinitis. Phytother Res. 2009 Jul; 23(7):920-6
12. Schapowal A. Randomised controlled trial of butterbur and cetirizine for treating seasonal allergic rhinitis. BMJ 2002; 324:144.
13. Bielory L, Heimall J. Review of complementary and alternative medicine in treatment of ocular allergies. Curr Opin Allergy Clin Immunol. 2003 Oct; 3(5):395-9.
14. Van Breemen RB, Tao Y, Li W.Cyclo oxygenase-2 inhibitors in ginger (Zingiber officinalis). Fitoterapia. 2010; Sept 15.
15. Jurenka JS. Anti inflammatory properties of curcumin, a major constituent of *Curcuma longa*: a review of preclinical and clinical research. Aztern Med Rev.; 14(2):141-53.
16. Ammon HP. Boswellic acids in chronic inflammatory diseases. Planta Med. 2006 Oct; 72(12):1100-16.
17. Darshan S, Doreswamy R.Patented anti-inflammatory plant drug development from traditional medicine. Phytother Res.2004 May; 18(5):343-57.
18. Wojtowicz JC, et al. Pilot, Prospective, Randomized, Double-masked, Placebo-controlled Clinical Trial of an Omega-3 Supplement for Dry Eyes. Cornea. 2010 Oct 28.

19. Pinheiro MN Jr. et al. [Oral flaxseed oil (*Linum usitatissimum*) in the treatment for dry-eye Sjögren's syndrome patients]. Arg Bras Oftalmol. 2007 Jul-Aug; 70(4):649-55.
20. Szakiel A et al. Antibacterial and antiparasitic activity oleanolic acid and its glycosides isolated from marigold (*Calendula officinalis*). Planta Med. 2008 Nov; 74(14): 1709-15.
21. Aithal GP. Hepatotoxicity related to antirheumatic drugs. Nat Rev Rheumatol. 25.
22. Aloisi AM, et al. Chronic pain therapy and hypothalamic-pituitary-adrenal axis impairment. Psychoneuroendocrinology. 2011 Jan 20.
23. Town T. Inflammation, immunity, and Alzheimer's disease. CNS Neurol Disord Drug Targets. 2010 Apr; 9(2): 129-31.
24. Castellani ML, et al. Interrelationship between vitamins and cytokines in immunity.J Biol Regul Homeost Agents. 2010 Oct-Dec; 24(4):385-90.
25. Onishi A, et al. Pseudoaldosteronism with increased serum cortisol associated with pneumonia, hypouricemia, hypocalcemia, and hypophosphatemia. ClinNephrol. 2010 Nov; 74(5):403-8.
26. Yang H, et al. Green tea Polyphenols as Proteasome Inhibitors: Implication in Chemoprevention. Curr Cancer Drug Targets. 2011 Jan 19.
27. Sharma PR, et al. Anticancer activity of an essential oil from *Cymbopogon flexuosus*. Chem Biol Interact. 2009 May 15; 179(2-3):160-8.
28. Ionkova I, Momekov G, Proksch P. Effect of cycloartane saponins from hairy roots of *Astragalus membranaceus* Bge., on human tumor cell targets. Fitotherapia. 2010 Jul; 81(5):447-51.
29. Cerella C, et al. Chemical Properties and Mechanisms Determining the Anti-Cancer Action of Garlic-Derived Organic Sulfur Compounds. Anticancer Agents Med Chem. 2011 Jan 26.
30. Amara AA, El-Masry MH, Bogdady HH. Pak J Plant crude extracts could be the solution: extracts showing in vivo antitumorigenic activity. Pharm Sci. 2008 Apr; 21(2):159-71.

31. Nerbass FB, et al.Effects of massage therapy on sleep quality after coronary artery bypass graft surgery. Clinics (Sao Paulo).2010; 65(11):1105-10.
32. Adams GR, et al. Exercise and leukocyte interchange among central circulation, lung, spleen, and muscle. Brain Behav Immun. 2011 Jan 14.
33. Zielinski MR, Krueger JM. Sleep and innate immunity. Front Biosci Schol Ed.). 2011 Jan 1; 3:632-42.
34. Salzman MB, Smith EM, Koo C. Excessive oral zinc supplementation.J Pediatr Hematol Oncol.2002 Oct;24(7):582-4.
35. Coussens LM, Werb Z. Inflammation and cancer. Nature. 2002 Dec 19-26; 420(6917):860-7.
36. Sharma M, et al. The potential use of Echinacea in acne: control of *Propionibacterium acnes* growth and inflammation. Phytother Res. 2010 Sep 9.
37. Barrett B, et al. Echinacea for treating the common cold: a randomized trial. Ann Intern Med. 2010 Dec 21; 153(12):769-77.
38. Dkhi MA, et al. Anticoccidial andf anti-inflammatory activity of garlic in muri Eimeria papillata infections. Vet Parasitol. 2011 Jan 10; 175(1-2):66-72.
39. Ban JO, et al. Anti-inflammatory and arthritic effects of thiacremonone, a novel sulfur compound isolated from garlic via inhibition of kappaB. Arthritis Res Ther. 2009; 11(5):R145.
40. Lee SH, et al. In vitro effects of plant and mushroom extracts on immunological function of chicken lymphocytes and macrophages. Br Poult Sci. 2010 Apr; 51(2):213-21.
41. Kawai K, et al. Catechin inhibits adhesion and migration of peripheral blood B cells by blocking CD11b. Immunopharmacol Immunotoxicol. 2010 Oct 11.
42. Monroe M, et al.Enhancement of phagocytic activity of macrophage-like cells with a crude polysaccharide derived from green tea (*Camellia sinensis*) extract. Biosci Biotechnol Biochem. 2010; 74(6):1306-8.
43. Rehman J, et al. Increased production of antigen-specific immunoglobulins G and M following in vivo treatment with

medicinal plants *Echinacea angustifolia* and *Hydrastis Canadensis.* Immunol Lett. 1999 jun 1; 68(2-3):391-5.

44. Carrasco FR, et al. Immunomodulatory activity of *Zingiber officinale* Roscoe, *Salvia officinalis* L. and *Syzygium aromaticum* L. essential oils: evidence for humor-and cell-mediated responses. J Pharm Pharmacol. 2009 Jul; 61(7):961-7.
45. Jang HI, Shin HM. Wild panax ginseng (Panax ginseng C.A.Meyer) protects against methotrexate- induced cell regression by enhancing the immune response in RAW 264.7 macrophages. Am J Chin Med. 2010; 38(5):949-60.
46. Li S, et al. Defective phagocytosis of apoptotic cells by macrophages in Atherosclerotic lesions of ob/ob mice and reversal by fish oil diet. Circ Res.2009 Nov 20;105(11):1072-82.
47. Cao H, Urban JF Jr, Anderson RA. Cinnamon polyphenol extract affects immune responses by regulating anti- and proinflammatory and glucose transporter gene expression in mouse macrophages. J Nutr.2008 May; 138(5):833-40.
48. Liu QY, Yao TM,Zhang SW, Sheng ZY. Astragalus polysaccharides regulate T cell-mediated immunity via CD11c(high)CD45RB(low) DCs in vitro. J Ethnopharmacol. 2010 Jul 8.
49. Groom SN, Johns T, Oldfield PR.The potency of immunomodulatory herbs may be primarily dependent upon macrophage activation. J Med Food. 2007 Mar; 10(1):73-9.
50. Zhang XY, et al. Proanthocyanidin from grape seeds potentiates anti-tumor activity of doxorubicin via immunomodulatory mechanism. Int Immunopharmacol. 2005 Jul: 5(7-8):1247-57.
51. Kim HN, et al. Vitamin C down-regulates VEGF production in B16F10 murine melanoma cells via the suppression of p42/44 MAPK activation. J Cell Biochem. 2010 Dec 29.
52. Harikrishnan R, et al. Immunomodulatory effect of soium alginate enriched diet in kelp grouper Epinephelus brneus against Streptococcus iniae. Fish Shellfish Immunol. 2010 Dec 3.
53. Harikrishnan R, et al. Protective effect of herbal and probiotics enriched diet on haematological and immunity status of

Oplegnathus fasciatus (Temminck & Schlegel) against Edwardsiella tarda. Fish Shellfish Immunol. 2011 Jan 24.

54. Ringsdorf WM Jr, Cheraskin E. Vitamin C & Wound Healing: Oral Surg Oral Med Oral Pathol. 1982 Mar; 53(3):231-6.
55. Henkin RI. Zinc in Wound Healing. N Engl J Med. Sept 1974; 291:675-76.
56. Harkenson KD, et al. Omega-3 fatty acids enhance ligament fibroblast collagen formation in association with changes in interleukin-6 production. Proc Soc Exp Biol Med. 2000 Jan; 223(1):88-95.
57. McDaniel JC, et al. Omega-3 fatty acids effect on wound healing. Wound Repair Regen. 2008 May-Jun; 16(3):337-45.
58. Ejaz S, et al. Effect of aged garlic extract on wound healing: a new frontier in wound management. Drug Chem Toxicol. 2009; 32(3):191-203.
59. Chithra P, Sajithlal GB, Chandrakasan G. Influence of aloe vera on the healing of dermal wounds in diabetic rats. J Ethnopharmacol. 1998 Jan; 59(3):195-201.
60. Teoh SL, Latiff AA, Das S.The effect of topical extract of Mormordica charantia (bitter gourd) on wound healing in nondiabetic rats and in rats with diabetes induced by streptozotocin. Clin Exp Dermatol. 2009 Oct; 34(7):815-22.

The Toxic Eye

Case Scenario One: Your patient is a 73-year-old male who has difficulty ambulating even with a cane and looks older than his stated age. The patient is a heavy smoker with a daily alcohol intake that often exceeds normal limits. He is disheveled and malnourished, and his wife insists her husband will not listen to anything she suggests about his health. With visually significant cataracts (20/200 and 20/400) in both eyes and high intraocular pressures (IOP 27 and 28 mmHg), there is no previous history of treatment. After a month of attempted nutritional rehabilitation and IOP control, he undergoes successful cataract/IOL surgery in the left eye, with minimal improvement due to optic nerve pallor, cupping, and poor retinal circulation. He refuses to change his debilitating habits and misses all follow-up appointments until one year later. The operated eye is No Light Perception and the fellow eye has Hand Motion Vision with corneal edema, acute uveitis, hypermature cataract with probable phacoanaphylaxis, IOP greater than 40 mmHg. After all this, he refuses surgery and asks defiantly, "Why can't I see?"

One of the most overlooked causes of a poor outcome from both medical and surgical treatments is the effects of toxins on the eye. In a body full of toxins, the eye will exhibit signs of the same toxicity given time and accumulation. The results will often lead to autoimmune and neurodegenerative diseases. The health status of the preoperative body will be closely related to the surgical outcome of the eye.

Despite advances in modern medicine, social, economic, medical, and ecological causes of toxicity, each continue to play a significant role in health issues; this includes the profound influence of poverty, malnutrition, dysfunctional nutrition, stress, and toxin abuse. Exposure to environmental toxins, accessibility to health care, neglect of preventive measures, and our culture's heavy reliance on antibiotics and steroids are mere factors which have led to the compromise of the immune system and ultimately to cellular, tissue, and organ damage. An increasing internal susceptibility to toxins, a proliferation of pathogenic microorganisms and an unstable equilibrium between clinical inflammatory and immunocompetent cells often leads to acute and chronic inflammation. This is often manifested in autoimmune and neurodegenerative diseases like Alzheimer's, multiple sclerosis, autism, Leber's optic neuropathy, and Parkinson's, in which mitochondrial dysfunction, oxidative stress, excitotoxicity, and neuroinflammation are regarded as the prevailing processes involved. (1) Prolonged exposure to air pollution is associated with narrower diameters of retinal blood vessels and subclinical cardiovascular disease in older individuals. (2)

Mechanism of Toxicity:

Toxins in the blood stream and at the tissue levels interfere with the transfer factor in the T-killer cells, which stimulates cell-mediated immunity. This leads to activation of immunocytokine synthesis, which results in cell-by-cell apoptosis (programmed cell death). At the cellular level, toxins block the mitochondrial oxidative phosphorylation pathways.

Toxins gain access to the blood stream and fluids of the eye by direct external contact (chemicals and pollution) to the conjunctiva and through the cornea. As the result of ingestion and skin and mucous membrane absorption, internal distribution of toxins travels into and through the blood stream. This may result in lens sclerosis (cataracts), like those resulting from prolonged use of steroids, and direct damage to the cornea, optic nerve, and retinal cells, such as from amiodarone (keratopathy) and hydroxychloroquine (retinopathy). (3) (4) In regard to the more common ocular conditions of glaucoma, diabetic retinopathy, and macular degeneration, the effects of toxicity are just being explored. The fact that 93 percent of Americans test positive for exposure to Bisphenol A (detrimental effects on neuronal differentiation and brain neurogenesis) should be a red flag that many of our most common disease entities may have some connection with toxicity. (5)(6) More everyday toxins like traffic pollutants (diesel exhaust particles) and cigarette smoke though exerting direct damage on their own, may cause additional destruction by enhancing cell sensitivity to other allergens, which leads to synthesis of more proinflammatory mediators. (7)

The effects of toxins are cumulative and dose related.

Skin (direct contact)	Mucous membranes	Lungs
Eye (conjunctiva, cornea)	Stomach, intestines	Placenta (mother to child)

Table 1: Site of Action:

External toxins may be absorbed directly through the skin and mucous membranes, or inhaled and absorbed through the lungs. Of the drain cleaners (alkalis), those with ammonia (NH3) most rapidly penetrate the eye and damage the cornea. Anhydrous ammonia appears to be the most dangerous. These types of ammonias are also found in some fertilizers and dishwasher gel packs. Handwashing and avoiding contact with the eyes is an important deterent when handling these materials. Household cleaners contain hypochlorous acid (HOCl), which releases chlorine when exposed to water. In swimming pools, when urea is added to this mixture, a strong eye irritant, which causes punctuate erosions and corneal edema is produced. Automobile fluids (hydrocarbons) can cause major injuries as well as hallucinations and abnormal visual evoked response, through the heat and pressure inhalation of leaded gas. The fluoride in wheel cleaners can penetrate the skin. Detergents like the preservative benzalkonium chloride, found in many ocular medications, can be harmful to the cornea and conjunctiva. Alcohols (20–40 percent) are used to remove the corneal epithelium in surgery. Harmful cyanoacryclates (CH2C(CN)COOCH3) are found in the Krazy Glue sometimes mistaken for eyedrops.Pesticides and herbicides contain methylmercury, which can leach into our fruits and vegetables and lead to conjunctivitis, miosis, accommodative spasm, and neurodegeneration. DEET (N, N-diethyl-3-methylbenzamide) in insect repellant, allethin, and permethin in tick repellant, and organophosphates and glycophosphates in weed killer can cause cholinergic side effects. Lachrymators like capsaicin (pepper spray) and chloroacetophenone (mace) are created for their ability to cause damage.

Cigarette smoke is perhaps the most common toxic irritant of all.

Drain cleaners	Household cleaners	Industrial cleaners	Tonometer cleaners	Insect repellant	Magnesium hydroxide
Lye soap	Wheel cleaners	Hydrofluori c acid	Hand cleaners	Weed killer	Alkaline batteries
Chlorine	Fireworks	Sulfuric acid	Crazy glue	Permethin	
Biodiesel s	Diesel	Alcohol	Pesticides	Brake fluid	
Cement	Gasoline	Methanol	Methylmercur y	Organophosphate	
Fertilizers	Detergents	Cosmetics	DEET	Antiseptics	

Table 2. External Chemicals Toxic to the Eye:

Methylmercury is a byproduct of the manufacture of acetaldehyde in pesticides and the burning of fossil fuels and is the one most likely to be discharged into marshes and streams. Seventy-five percent of food manufacturers in the USA use pesticides. They have widespread use in parks, playgrounds, schools, homes, and golf courses.

Wash fruits and vegetables well before eating.

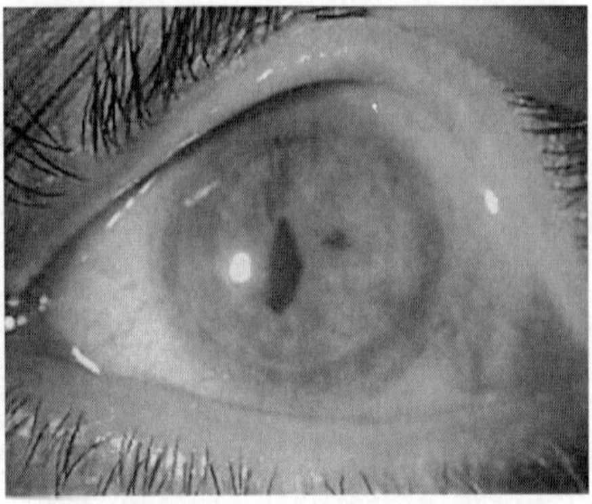

cigarette toxicity in an immune-compromised
eye 5 years after corneal transplant

Internal toxins include medications, heavy metals, pesticides/herbicides, food additives, and drugs. *Medications* with known adverse effects on the optic nerve include the following: Barbitols, antibiotics like chloramphenicol and clindamycin; the measles, mumps, and rubella vaccine; naproxen, chlorpropramide and tolbutamide, isoniazid and ethambutol, the sulfur derivatives, iodide and iodine solutions, interferon alpha, beta and gamma, tetanus immune globulin and toxoid, and vincristine and vinblastine can all cause retrobulbar and optic neuritis. Hydroxychloroquine has been associated with bull's eye maculopathy in which vision loss may be progressive and irreversible even if the medication is discontinued. Anticoagulants like clopidogel bisulfate have been associated with intraocular hemorrhage. (8) Amiodarone, used in the treatment of arrhythmias, can cause verticillate keratopathy and optic neuropathy. (9)

Heavy metals are found mainly in fumes and solvents, which are components of common household devices. Mercury is the most common, but it is only the third most hazardous of the heavy metal toxins behind arsenic (number one) and lead (number two). Entry of this toxin into the bloodstream is through the lungs or intestines, and it courses to the nervous system and organs, especially kidneys and brain, where the inhibition of protein synthesis and selenium metabolism, activation of cell membrane damaging enzymes, and the disruption of energy production in the mitochondria of nerve and immune cells occurs. Methylmercury has a particular affinity for sulfhydryl, amine, phosphoryl and carboxyl groups, which allows it to adhere to internal surfaces of the cell. It is better diagnosed by hair analysis than by blood testing. Symptoms of the eye may take years to appear and manifest as dizziness and headaches, memory loss, and constriction of visual fields.

One of the best-known vehicles for heavy metal access into the body is dental amalgams, which contain the standard of 50 percent Hg, 35 percent Ag, 13 percent Sn and 2 percent Cu. The mercury may leach out over a lifetime of chewing. Broken thermometers; fungicides and pesticides used to treat grains and seeds; waste incinerators, cement kilns, and coal combustors; vaccines preserved in thimerosal; contact lens' solutions and fluorescent bulbs all release mercury vapors. The most common mercury medicines are laxatives, organic mercurial diuretics, cathartics, and antihelminthics. Ocean fish are also high in mercury and the bigger the fish, like shark and kingfish, the more the mercury content.

Methlymercury induces neurotoxicity and cell death by blocking pathways involved with lysozymes and calcium-dependent proteases, which mainly affect the optic nerve and retina. (10) (11)

In the cosmetics industry, mercury is an added ingredient intended to contain and control the prevention of bacterial growth. The FDA allows sixty-five ppm, but many eye make-ups contain over 650 ppm in the form of mercurous chloride.

The aluminum in processed cheeses, teas with lemon, pancakes, biscuits, foods with baking powder, cookware, certain medications, vaccinations, processed fruit juices, and in gaseous fluoride exhausts in factories, can cause allergic ocular symptoms in hypersensitive individuals. (12)

Dental amalgams	Chlorine products	Fluorescent bulbs	Floor waxes	Fabric softeners
Thermometers	Vaccines	Mirrors	Tattoo dyes	Cosmetics
Incinerators	Medicines	Felt hats	Ocean fish	Fuel exhausts

Table 3. Products with Heavy Metals Toxic to the Eye:

Excitoxicity:

Of the food additives, monosodium glutamate (MSG) is the most important factor for the increase in obesity, inflammatory diseases, and type 2 diabetes over the last thirty years. It is a hydrolyzed vegetable protein, which is the *secret spice* that gives that addictive flavoring to many of our high-calorie food products. As an excitotoxin, MSG is an excitatory neurotransmitter that binds to the receptors of nerve cells and allows high levels of calcium ions to flood the cell; this in turn, activates enzymes such as phospholipases, endonucleases, and proteases, which damage cell membranes and result in ischemic neurodegeneration. (13) Ischemic retinopathy plays a major role in the pathophysiology of diabetic retinopathy, glaucoma, anterior ischemic optic neuropathy, and age-related macular degeneration. (14) MSG increases insulin production in the pancreas, which increases diabetic retinopathy.

Aspartame—which is methanol and aspartate—transforms to formaldehyde and formic acid and creates a metabolic acidosis in the bloodstream; it is associated with autoimmune neurodegenerative diseases like autism, multiple sclerosis, Parkinson's, Alzheimer's, systemic lupus, fibromyalgia, and leukemic cancers, all of which exhibit signs of retinal ischemia at some point in their progression. Calorie-free artificial sweeteners increase the concentration of aspartatic acid and phenylalanine, both of which are neurotoxic. (15) (16)

In glaucoma, high intraocular pressure reduces blood flow to the eye, which in turn triggers the release of the excitatory neurotoxin glutamate into the vitreous. (17) In diabetics, injured nerve cells and glial cells release glutamate, which causes further destruction to nerve cells, particularly the astrocytes.

A Power Lunch: Soup, sandwich, Diet Coke, chips, canned food, packaged meat, and salad dressing.

The most commonly abused drugs are nicotine (C23H27N) and alcohol (C2H6O). Cigarettes are comprised of vast quantities of toxic chemicals of which 98 percent are tars and a mere 2 percent is tobacco. The average cigarette has 1 mg of nicotine plus wood alcohol and methyl alcohol. They contain the same alkaloids found in the nightshade family (Solanaceae) of datura and belladonna plants. These alkaloids contain poisons (tropanes), which are metabolized in the liver into cotinine and acrolein; both substances irreversibly bind to DNA in cells, thus causing mutations and cancer. Tobacco use is associated with vitamin C deficiency and excessive alcohol use is associated with alpha-linoleic acid deficiency. Both conditions are associated with age related degenerative maculopathy. (18) Chronic accumulation of cigarette smoke in the lens is associated with oxidative damage to the lens, and such damage results in nuclear cataract. (19) Many eye symptoms are related to the vasoconstriction of retinal vessels and consist of amaurosis and visual field constriction. The cyanides released are associated with a vitamin B12 deficiency, which causes damage to nerve cells and blood vessel linings. With prolonged exposure to the toxins found in cigarettes, nicotinic receptors in the central nervous system (CNS) that normally receive acetylcholine act as dopaminergic systems associated with addictive properties which activate and desensitize blood vessels. This effect often leads to retinal artery thrombosis and visual loss. In the *Beaver Dam Eye Study*, there was an increase in the cumulative incidence and progression of macular degeneration in smokers over age fifty. (20) (21)

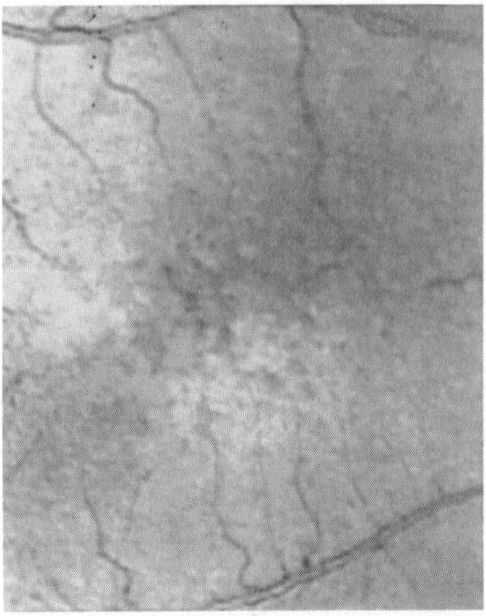

toxic maculopathy

Streptomycin	Hydroquinolone s	Disulfram	Lead	Nickel
Linezolid	Alcohol	Glutamate	Arsenic	Vaccines (live)
Chloramphenico l	Nicotine /tars	Aspartic acid	Cadmium	Minoxidil
Isoniazid Ethambutol	Ethyl glycol (antifreeze)	Cyanide	Mercury	Clopidogrel

Table 4: Internal Chemicals Toxic to the Eye:

Eye Symptoms of Toxicity:

Many medications can cause optic neuropathy, hemorrhage, optic atrophy, and optic edema. Pesticides and herbicides can lead to burning, conjunctivitis, accommodative spasm, and neurodegeneration. Heavy metals can cause dizziness, headache, constricted visual fields, and neurodegeneration. Food additives can cause blurred vision, memory loss, tinnitus, neurodegeneration, and blindness. Drug abuse can cause dilated pupils, conjunctival irritation, dry eyes, and cataract. The general symptoms of toxicity include red-green dyschromatopsia, monocular then bilateral, sluggish pupils, hyperemic discs, then pallor; +/- splinter hemorrhages; late papillomacular bundle dropout and temporal pallor, then optic atrophy; and painless, acute then chronic, gradual then progressive dimming of vision.

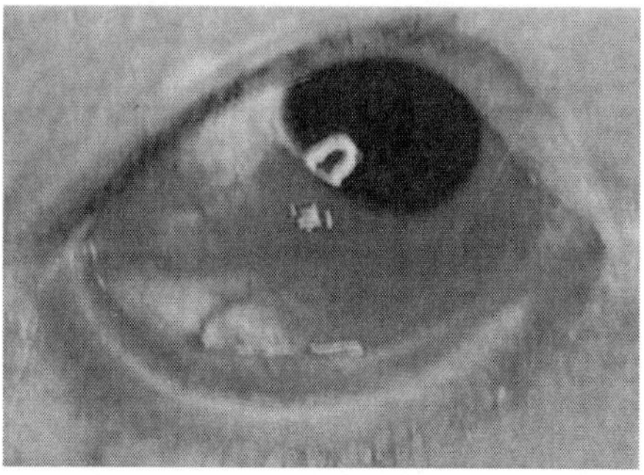

Figure 3. Conjunctival hemorrhage in a patient taking oral blood thinners

Clonidine	Thioridazine	Plaquenil	Venlafaxine
Fenfluramine	Mirtazapine	Simvastatin	antihistamines
oral hypoglycemics	antidepressants	birth control pills	sulfa drugs
corticosteroids	antispasmodics	tranquilizers	NSAIDS

Table 5. Drugs Associated with Retina and Optic Nerve Damage

Case Scenario Two: In the emergency room, a 34-year-old male presented with barely light perception in both eyes due to gradual visual loss over a six-month period. His blood sugar was 375 mg percent and a fundus examination revealed a retinopathy was not commensurate with the extent of visual loss. He had no family history of diabetes and no previous diagnosis of eye disease. The patient owned and managed a neighborhood grocery specializing in exotic foods, and admitted to acquiring a daily habit over the past five years of drinking up to one case of Coca-Cola and smoking up to two packs of cigarettes daily. Laser pan photocoagulation and anti-VEGF were to no avail. Within another six months, he became NLP (No Light Perception).

Toxins -> retinal ischemia + inflammation -> cataract, diabetic retinopathy, optic neuropathy, glaucoma and often, vision inconsistent with findings.

Tropical Optic Neuropathy:

Jamaican bush tea can be any of over 200 varieties, all of which contain high quantities of the neurotoxic cassava plant containing the cyanoglucosides, linamarin and lotaustralin, which are hydrolysed to acetonecyanohydrin and cyanide. (22)

In Guadeloupe, an abnormally high incidence of atypical Parkinson's resembling progressive supranuclear palsy (PSP) associated with ingestion of soursop (Annona muricata) fruit and leaf tea has been reported. (23)

Other plants with adverse ocular effects are manchineel, oleander, ortiga, nutmeg, castor oil, avocado leaves, soursop, gladiola, dumbcane, trumpet flower, nutmeg, amanita mushrooms, water hemlock, and artemesia.

Obtaining a history of toxin exposure, occupational background, and use of herbal preparations is mandatory in any medical examination.

Diagnostic testing:

Magnetic Resonance Imaging (MRI) can identify the site of optic nerve damage. Blood testing for heavy metals, methanol levels (blood > 50 mg/ml) or gas chromatography (>0.5-1.0 mg/kg.), vitamin B12 levels less than 200 pg/ml in adults is below normal. Vitamin D deficiency is associated with heart disease and macular degeneration. (24) C-reactive protein levels greater than 2.4 mg/l indicate the presence of inflammation. Homocysteine levels greater than 14 micromoles/l indicates cardiovascular damage, especially to the inner lining of arterioles. Color testing with Farnsworth and Ishihara plates can identify the presence of dyschromatopsia. Fluorescein angiography can highlight defects in the retinal vasculature. Hair analysis is available for mercury levels.

Complimentary Treatment:

The best treatment is *avoidance*, closely followed by prevention by maintaining a healthy immune system. Skin, liver, intestines, and kidneys are excellent natural detoxification centers when functioning properly. Heavy metals like dental amalgam fillings can be replaced with porcelain or similar nonreactive material. Beware of body cleansers like footbaths and pads, as they are usually bogus. Detoxification with natural products like lemon, olive oil apple cider vinegar, milk thistle, dandelion, garlic, onions, oat bran, antioxidants, lots of fiber, and pure water on a regular basis is good. Beware of long-term fasting as essential vitamins and minerals may also be lost. Omega-3 can reduce and improve the effects of oxidative stress in the kidneys. Chelation with EDTA (ethylenediaminetetraacetic acid) binds some heavy metals and removes them from the body via the urinary tract. Selenium binds to methymercury and neutralizes the toxic effects. (25) (26) (27) Malate and creatine pyruvate bind to aluminum and block its absorption. Silymarin (milk thistle), curcumin (turmeric), quercetin, and kelp protect neurons and neutralize toxic effects of most heavy metals.

It is important to note that the perspiration, which results from regular physical activity (exercise), contains high levels of excreted toxins. Exercise also increases the body's immune system defenses.

References for Chapter Three:

1. Barnum CJ, Tansey MG. Modeling neuroinflammatory pathogenesis of Parkinson's disease. Prog Brain Res. 2010; 184:113-32
2. Adar SD, et al. Air Pollution and microvasculature: a cross-sectional assessment of in vivo retinal images in the population-based multi-ethnic study of atherosclerosis (MESA). PLos Med. 2010 Nov 30; (11):e100037

3. Erdurmus M, et al. Amiodarone-induced keratopathy:full thickness corneal involvement. Eye Contact Lens. 2008 Mar; 34(2): 131-2
4. Hanna B, et al. Retinal toxicity secondary to Plaquenil therapy. Optometry. 2008 Feb; 79(2):90-4.
5. Calafat AM, et al. Exposure of the U.S. population to bisphenol A and 4-tertiary octyphenol: 2003-2004. Environ Health Perspect. 2008 Jan; 116(1):39-44.
6. Kim K, et al. Potencies of bisphenol A on neuronal differentiation and hippocampal neurogenesis. J Toxicol Environ Health A. 2009; 72(21-22): 1343-51.
7. Davies RJ, Rusznak C, Devalia JL.Why is allergy increasing?—environmental factors. Clin Exp Allergy.1998 Dec; 28 Suppl 6:8-14.
8. Kiernan DF, et al. Epidemiology of the association between anticoagulants and intraocular hemorrhage in patients with neovascular age-related macular degeneration. Retina. 2010 Nov-Dec; 30(10): 1573-8.
9. Speicher MA, Goldman MH, Chrousos GA. Amiodarone optic neuropathy without disc edema. J Neuroophthalmol. 2000 Sep; 20(3): 171-2.
10. Ceccatelli S, Daré E,Moors M. Methylmercury-induced neurotoxicity and apoptosis. Chem Biol Interact. 2010 Nov 5; 188(2):301-8.
11. Myers GJ, Davidson PW, Strain JJ. Nutrient and methylmercury exposure from consuming fish. J Nutr. 2007 Dec; 137(12):2805-8.
12. Larsson B, Karlsson JE, Nielsen J. Respiratory and ocular symptoms in workers exposed to potassium aluminum-tetrafluoride soldering flux. Int Arch Occup Environ Health. 2007 Jul; 80(7):627-33.
13. Roman-Ramos R, et al.Monosodium Glutamate Neonatal Intoxication Associated with Obesity in Adult Stage is Characterized by Chronic Inflammation and Increased mRNA Expression of Peroxisome Proliferation Activated Receptors in Mice. Basic Clin Pharmacol Toxicol. 2011 Jan 3.
14. Neroev VV, Zueva, Kalamkarov GR. Molecular mechanisms of retinal ischemia. Vestn Oftalmol. 2010 May-Jun; 126(3): 59-64.

15. Whitehouse CR, Boullata J, McCauley LA.The potential toxicity of artificial sweeteners. AAOHN J. 2008 Jun; 56(6): 251-9.
16. O'Connell ED, et al. Diet and risk factors for age-related maculopathy. Am J Clin Nutr. 2008 Mar; 87(3): 712-22.
17. Dreyer EB, et al. Elevated glutamate levels in the vitreous body of humans and monkeys with glaucoma. Arch Ophthalmol. 1996 Mar; 114(3): 299-306.
18. Shalini VK, et al. Oxidative damage to the eye lens caused by cigarette smoke and fuel smoke condensates. Indian J Biochem Biophys. 1994 Aug; 31(4):261-6.
19. Klein R, et al. Further observations on the association between smoking and the long-term incidence and progression of age-related macular degeneration: the Beaver Dam Eye Study. Arch Ophthalmol. 2008 Jan; 126(1):115-21.
20. Klein R, Klein BE, Moss SE. Relation of smoking to the incidence of age-related maculopathy. The Beaver Dam Eye Study. Am J Epidemiol. 1998 Jan 15; 147(2):103-10.
21. Klein R, et al. The Beaver Dam Eye Study: the relation of age-related maculopathy to smoking. Am J Epidemiol. 1993 Jan 15; 137(2): 190-200.
22. Nambisan B. Strategies for elimination of cyanogens from cassava for reducing toxicity and improving food safety. Food Chem Toxicol. 2011 Mar; 49(3):690-3.
23. Lannuzel A, et al. Atypical parkinsonism in Guadeloupe: a common risk factor for two closely related phenotypes? Brain. 2007 Mar; 130(Pt 3):816-27.
24. Mascitelli L, et al.Macular degeneration, heart disease and vitamin D. Ophthalmol. 2010 Jan; 117(1):194
25. Lauretani F, et al. Omega-3 and renal function in older adults. Curr Pharm Des. 2009; 15(36): 4149-56.
26. Zhang M, et al. Topical metal chelation therapy ameliorates oxidation-induced toxicity in diabetic cataract. J Toxicol Environ Health A. 2011 Jan; 74(6): 380-91.
27. Berry MJ, Ralston NV.Mercury toxicity and the mitigating role of selenium. Ecohealth. 2008 Dec; 5(4):456-9.

Internal Diseases

Case Scenario One: "I am 59 years old and my doctor says I have early cataracts. My vision is slightly blurred at times, but I can see the 20/25 lines on the charts and can read the small print pretty easily when the lighting is good. I prefer not to have surgery. What else can I do to prevent them from getting worse too quickly?"

"Long-term supplementary high-dose vitamin C and vitamin E used alone or in conjunction, had no appreciable positive or negative effects on rates of age-related cataract in middle-aged and older men, a large study showed." (1)

"There is no concrete evidence for or against the prevention or reversal of cataracts using medications or supplements." (2)

"High plasma levels of retinol are associated with lower risk of cataracts." (3)

There is evidence for and against the use of complementary measures that may be effective in the approach to the medical treatment of cataracts. When considering the structure of the studies being conducted, the following approaches are reasonable: Evidence suggests there is no harm done by using prevention methods. The use of supplements is supported by logic and the possibility that the placebo effect may be real.

In reality, cataract epidemiological studies are very difficult to perform. Preventive measures in animal studies have shown promising results that have so far not been duplicated in human epidemiological studies. It is difficult to amass 11,000 plus men and women and expect all their crystalline lenses to be at the same level of development. The subjects are not going to fall into the same categories, and over a five- to ten-year period, they will not all exhibit the same behavior on a consistent basis. There is no absolute control in most human studies due to the very nature of the subjects.

If you know the pathogenesis and pathophysiology of a condition, then the possible mechanisms required for prevention and treatment can be addressed. It is generally agreed that the formation of cataracts is based on a combination of environment, hereditary factors, diet, age, and lifestyle risk factors. Vitamin E is an antioxidant found in lens fibers that may slow cataract formation by reducing lipid peroxidation and stabilizing cell membranes. Vitamin C is an antioxidant in the aqueous compartments of lens membranes that may protect lens proteases from photooxidative destruction. Cataract formation is gradual and appears to be associated with the presence of oxidative stress, increased lipid peroxide and glycolated protein, increased free radicals, reduced glutathione and superoxide scavenging activity, and breakdown in the barrier function of cell membranes, as evidenced with cigarette smoking, UV radiation exposure, and poor nutrition, all of which reduce the levels of antioxidants in the lens and promote cataract formation. (4) (5) The presence of high glucose levels (diabetes mellitus), inflammation, and long-term use of systemic and topical steroids are also associated risk factors for cataract formation. (6) (7) (8) (9) (10)

Not smoking, reducing exposure to UV radiation, and maintaining adequate nutritional levels of antioxidants are logical, inexpensive, and possibly effective strategies of delaying the onset or reducing the progression of age-related cataracts. (11)

The use of topical or systemic supplements specifically designed for and targeting age related cataracts continues to be controversial. Topical N-acetylcarnosine, 5-S-GAD, bendazac-lysine and cineraria maritima have been shown to reduce cataract formation in human and animal studies. (12) (13) (14) (15) (16) In my experience, using sulfacetamide drops in patients with early-age-related cataract accomplishes similar results in delaying the formation of visually significant cataract. Adding lifestyle awareness and implementation of nutritional factors, the placebo effect may well be active in these cases. The results are real and can be duplicated in a variable population and warrant further investigation perhaps with smaller, better-controlled human studies. (17) (18) (19)

As long as doctors promote surgery as the only treatment for cataracts, it is unlikely that a therapeutic drug or definitive preventive measure to delay or reverse age-related cataracts will be accepted by all anytime soon. Though it is generally accepted that hard evidence for preventing or reversing cataracts is lacking and that there is little or no initiative for obtaining it, there are still reasonable actions that can be taken to *slow the progression*.

Complementary Daily Cataract Prevention Protocol:

Objective: Reduce oxidative stress and improve essential nutrients for proper lens metabolism

1. Avoid risky behavior: Smoking, excessive ultraviolet radiation exposure, long-term drugs (steroids), toxic medications, diabetes, diet high in saturated fats and fried foods, and deficient in antioxidants.
2. Antioxidants: Green leafy vegetables (Spinach leaf, broccoli, asparagus, kale, parsley, collards, plus onions, tomatoes, carrots—lightly cooked).
3. Supplements: Multivitamin with C (1000 mg), E (400 IU) and A (beta-carotene10,000 IU), selenium (200 micrograms), zinc (30), copper (2 mg), glutathione (50 mg), omega-3 fish oil; green tea; quercetin; turmeric (capsule or add powder to food as an anti-inflammatory and antioxidant)

4. Eyedrops: Cineraria maritima (silver ragwort), n-acetylcarnosine (NAC), or sulfacetamide 10 percent (or all three together) twice daily.

*This regimen is offered to every patient with early cataract formation and is accepted by 100 percent of them.

Selenium is an essential mineral found in Brazil nuts, tuna, cod, beef and poultry that is essential to glutathione synthesis. Glutathione is essential for lens metabolism and its absence leads to an increase in lens susceptibility to oxidative stress. (20) (21)

Green tea can be taken two or three times a day and its epigallocatechin gallate is a potent antioxidant and cell rejuvenator. (22)

Curcumin reduces free radical cataractogenesis through regulations in calcium metabolism. (23)

Sulfur compounds play a role in blocking the enzymes involved with cataract formation. (24)

"Observational data from the AREDS report no. 21 and the Longitudinal Study of Cataract suggest that use of a multivitamin with A, C, and E, may delay the progression of lens opacities." (25)

Mercury, lead, and cadmium (associated with smoking) are associated with increased risk of cataract formation. Detoxification on a regular basis will help reduce the concentration of these toxic metals. (26)

Complimentary measures focus on avoidance of detrimental habits (avoidable risk factors) and emphasize prevention, support, and maintenance of normal physiological health through good nutrition, early and frequent eye exams, regular physical activity, and healthy mindset. The primary objective is to neutralize or repair free radical damage as the main cause of tissue degeneration.

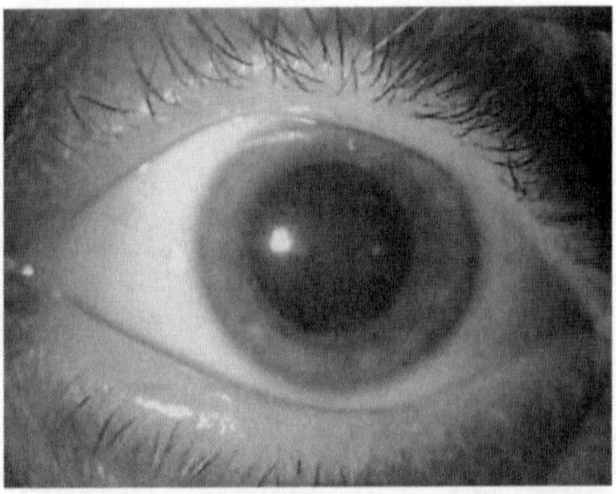

early age-related nuclear sclerotic cataract

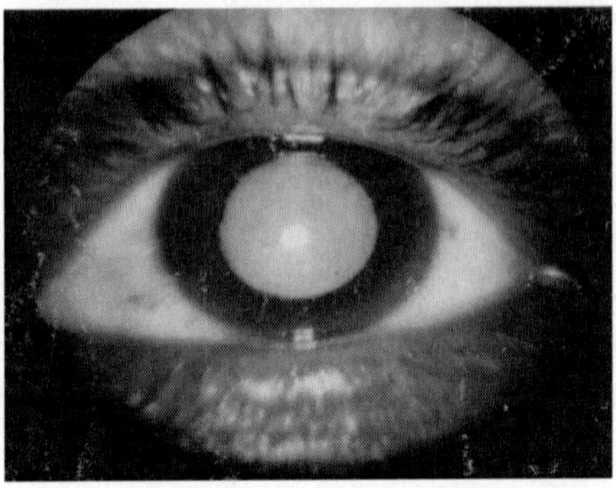

late hypermature cataract

It is better to start early (age forty) in modifying lifestyle and adopting a protocol of prevention to reduce the risk of rapid cataract formation. Early lens sclerosis responds more readily and positively than later more established sclerotic lenses.

Alcohol use has not been associated with cataract formation.

Case Scenario Two: A 34-year-old male of African Caribbean ancestry presents with intraocular pressures of 26 mmHg in right eye and 28 mmHg in the left, disc asymmetry and minimal cupping, normal visual fields, and a positive family history of glaucoma. He relates how his mother and paternal grandfather were blind, in spite of using eyedrops. While looking at his new prescriptions and reviewing his surgical options, he asks, "What else can I do to prevent or control glaucoma?"

A review of the causes of glaucoma can reveal possible avenues where complementary treatment could be of benefit in slowing the inevitable progression of glaucoma. The causes and progression of glaucomatous optic neuropathy are multifactorial. Hereditary risk factors, high intraocular pressure, low blood perfusion pressure, retinal ischemia, aging retinal vessels, glutamate excitotoxicity, altered immune response, and neurodegenerative factors all play a role in producing the characteristic visual field defects and eventual loss of vision through cell death. (27) (28)

"The Barbados Eye Studies" highlighted the roles of family history, higher intraocular pressure, and low blood perfusion pressure as high risk factors for glaucoma. (29)

The optic nerve appears to be susceptible to both high blood pressure and low blood pressure, as they both affect the perfusion pressure (OPP) and thus, the blood flow to the nerve. (30) Hypoxia and ischemia of the retina impair basal retinal and optic nerve metabolism, which leads to neovascularization and cell apoptosis. Ganglion cells are particularly susceptible. Cell acidosis, oxidative stress, excitotoxicity, and inflammation are also involved as trigger mechanisms and/or sequelae. (31) High intraocular pressure leads to the typical retinal nerve fiber layer deterioration seen in glaucoma. The fact that progressive visual field changes and neuronal cell loss can continue despite lowering of the intraocular pressure attests to the involvement and interplay of multiple mechanisms. (32) Glutamate and nitric oxide are found in excess in damaged neuronal cells. Neuroprotection or restoration of these cells may be accomplished with therapies that reduce or block these destructive substances. (33) The immune system provides a protective function for retinal neurons. Extremes and variations in intraocular pressure and blood pressure can lead to the neurodegeneration seen in glaucoma and implicate immunity as a major factor. (34) The contribution of toxic substances in the mechanisms of glaucoma is being considered as a major causal factor. Plasma levels of homocysteine are high in pseudoexfoliation glaucoma, and those of vitamin B6 were found to be elevated in normal tension and primary open-angle glaucoma groups. (35)

Though control of the intraocular pressure is a key factor in delaying or reducing the damaging effects of glaucoma, the research and data suggest that additional factors involving blood perfusion and neuronal cell integrity are involved. Ocular perfusion depends on perfusion pressure, vascular resistance and blood viscosity. Anything that helps regulate or normalize these physiologic parameters should improve blood flow to the optic nerve and retina and help with their preservation.

Glaucomatous Optic Neuropathy

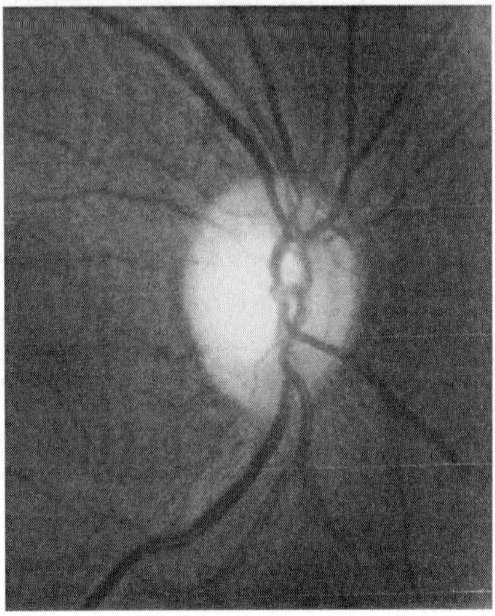

disc pallor with reduced blood perfusion

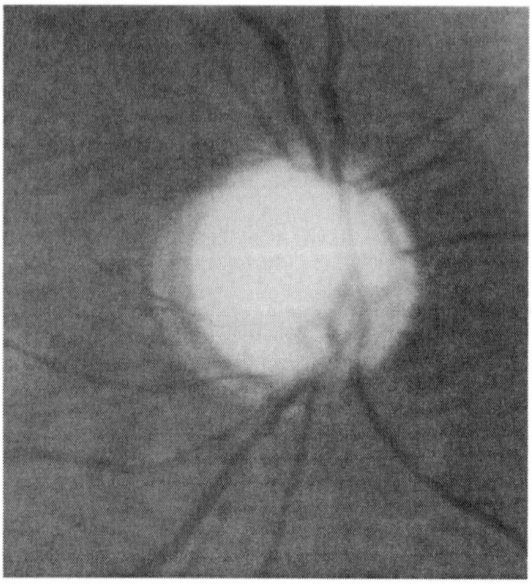

disc cupping with rim erosion

Recommended Complementary Daily Glaucoma Protocol:

Objective: Reduce oxidative stress; improve blood flow; protect blood vessel walls, optic nerve lining, and neuronal cells; regulate blood pressure; and control intraocular pressure

1. *Ginkgo biloba* (60 mg, 24 percent) as tea or capsules.
2. Coenzyme Q10 (ubiquinone) (100 mg).
3. Multivitamin with: ascorbic acid (1000 mg) and selenium (200 mcg).
4. Omega-3 fish oil (1000 mg in form of EPA and DHA).
5. Antioxidants (flavonoids) red wine, dark chocolate, coffee, tea, fruit, and colored vegetables with quercetin; bilberry and other berries.
6. Marijuana tea or drops (controversial).
7. Exercise (walk three days a week, minimum thirty minutes each day 1.5 miles, up to five times a week, forty minutes each for two miles.
8. Stress control.

A few studies show the neuroprotective effect and positive response of ocular blood flow to alcohol, *Ginkgo biloba*, and bilberry, but support is weak for their routine use. (36) Ginkgo biloba reduces and protects against inflammation, increases blood flow to small vessels, reduces vasospasm, reduces serum viscosity, inhibits platelet-activating factor, inhibits apoptosis, inhibits excitotoxicity, and improves central and peripheral blood flow. Though having no effect on intraocular pressure, *Ginkgo biloba* appeared to improve preexisting visual field changes in some patients with normal-tension glaucoma. It deserves further studies in the consideration of treatment for glaucomatous optic neuropathy. (37) (38) (39) Coenzyme Q10 in animal studies, offered retinal ganglion cell protection by the deactivation of excitotoxicity in the apoptosis mechanism and subsequent reduction of extracellular glutamate. (40) Preliminary studies have shown a relationship between ascorbic acid (Vitamin C) and selenium in normal tension and primary open-angle glaucoma subjects. (41) (42)

Omega-3 fish oil (docosanoids) reduces intraocular pressure by increasing aqueous outflow through improved outflow facility and reduced ocular rigidity. (43) (44)

Antioxidants with quercetin protect against the oxidative stress-induced glaucoma by activating specific NRF gene expression. (45) Polyphenolic compounds like tea, coffee, dark chocolate, and red wine reduce oxidative stress at the mitochondrial level. Coffee contains 3-methyl-1, 2-cyclopentanedione, which scavenges the axon-damaging peroxynitrite. The resveratrol in red wine inhibits the synthesis of the glial cell-activating compound, endothelin. Dark chocolate reduces blood pressure and improves vasorelaxation. (46) The anthocyanins in bilberries and blueberries are also beneficial in reducing age-related oxidative stress and improving neuronal function. (47)

The use of marijuana (*Cannabis sativa*) in glaucoma for its intraocular pressure-lowering effects has been controversial.

Inhalation has been discouraged by some clinicians because of its toxicological profile and side effects of postural hypotension, palpitations, tachycardia, and alterations in mental status. The mechanism of action appears to involve the decreased pressure perfusion of the ciliary body, as a result of the peripheral vasodilatory properties. The lowered blood pressure may further compromise the optic nerve. Topical delta 9-tetrahydrocannabinol administered either by inhalation or by oral capsules lowers IOP, but with concomitant, significant decreases in systolic blood pressure as well. Topical administration of marijuana drops has not been shown to lower IOP effectively. (48) (49) (50) (51) (52)

Both dynamic exercise and physical fitness have been associated with an acute decrease in intraocular pressure (IOP), as well as a lowered baseline IOP. Improvements in ocular blood flow and perfusion pressure may be the mechanisms involved. (53) (54)

Physical and emotional stress leads to increased plasma cortisol levels, which are associated with higher intraocular pressures and possible adrenal suppression mechanisms in glaucoma patients. (55) (56)

Other nutrients and botanicals showing some potential for complementary glaucoma treatment include lipoic acid, vitamin B12, magnesium, melatonin, forskolin (from *Coleus forskohlii*), and intramuscular injections of *Salvia miltiorrhiza*. (57)

Case Scenario Three: A 55-year-old obese African American female presents with blurred vision in both eyes which recently became worse. She has a history of established type 2 diabetes on oral hypoglycemics, hypertension on two antihypertensives, and hypercholesterolemia on statins. Her fasting blood glucose was 190 mg percent, her HbA1c was 8.3 percent, cholesterol was 230 mg/dl, and her sitting blood pressure was 145/90. She asks, "If I keep taking my medicine and my sugar goes down, will I still go blind from diabetes?"

This patient would definitely benefit from lifestyle changes, mainly diet and exercise, suited to improve control of diabetes and her other related systemic conditions. Blood sugar control may not be the only regulatory mechanism she needs to achieve better health.

Diabetes mellitus is a disease of the microvascular and macrovascular systems in which all organs are eventually rendered dysfunctional by elevated levels of blood glucose; it is caused by a combination of high caloric intake, poor utilization, and physical inactivity; it is a major health problem worldwide whose incidence appears to be increasing. Because it is characterized by disturbances of carbohydrate, lipid, and protein metabolism, many studies suggest that oxidative stress plays a significant role in the pathogenesis of diabetes mellitus. However, literary evidence suggests that there is no established benefit for the routine use of antioxidants in type 2 diabetes on the one hand and another review concludes there is evidence that nutritional supplements may be beneficial in the treatment or prevention in general. (58) (59) The pathogenesis of diabetes has multiple origins. Oxidative damage to the retinal mitochondria DNA stimulates the activation of matrix metalloproteinase-2, causing capillary cells to undergo apoptosis. Capillary endothelium dysfunction resulting from imbalances between vasoconstrictor and vasodilator substances leading to inflammatory, proliferative, and fibrotic processes that characterize progressive diabetic retinopathy. (60) (61)

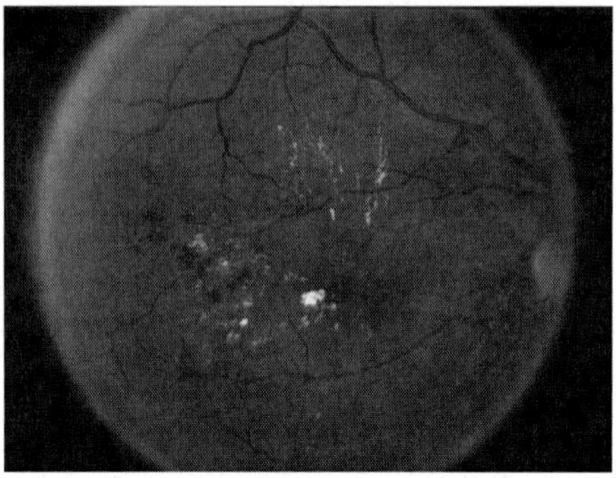

diabetic exudates & hemorrhages

With the increasing incidence and prevalence of diabetes mellitus, our treatment regimens through suppressive drugs may not be the answer to blood sugar control. Perhaps new strategies of treatment should be directed at the molecular and cellular causes and with simpler, wider ranging and more effective means. Integrative medicine enhances the therapeutic effects of hyperglycemia control, improved insulin resistance, glucose tolerance, pancreatic cell function, and lipid metabolism; it is a more complete approach.

*Complementary Daily Diabetes Mellitus Protocol **

Objective: Prevention of retinopathy by reducing insulin resistance, capillary fragility, autoimmunity, lipid peroxidation, decreasing viscosity, increasing blood flow.

Diet: Low-glycemic foods (Lentils, whole grains, beans, ...). magnesium-rich foods (spinach, broccoli, pumpkin seeds, fruit, nonfat dairy, lean meats, poultry, fish), omega-3 foods (cold-water fish, walnuts, freshly ground flaxseed), fruits and vegetables should be 50–60 percent of the diet. W*eight management,* eat smaller more frequent meals (five times a day), reduce starches (white rice) and sugars (processed, packaged foods), reduce saturated and transfats; use polyunsaturated and monounsaturated fats instead (30 percent of diet). Fiber should be the remaining 10–15 percent. Cholesterol at or below 200 mg/dl. Reducing fat and sugar improves cellular function, so that they become insulin sensitive instead of resistant. Fats in the bloodstream block the effectiveness of insulin.

Green leafy vegetables	Coenzyme Q10	Alpha lipoic acid	Omega-3 ffa (plant-based)	Magnesium rich foods
Onions	Garlic	Whole grains	Beans	Lentils
Chromium	Coffee	Soy products	Avocados	Cucumber
Vitamins C&E	Fiber	Quercetin	Vitamin D	DHEA

Table 1: Nutritional Supplements Beneficial to Type 2 Diabetes Mellitus.

*Support for nutritional supplementation as a main treatment in type 2 diabetes is a firm policy of the WHO and the world medical community.

Increased consumption of green leafy vegetables was associated with reduced incidence of type 2 diabetes (T2D). Lutein is a carotenoid present in large amounts in dark green vegetables. It reduced the formation of cross-links and chromosome instability in cells. (62) (63) (64) Experimental studies showed that alpha-lipoic acid (ALA), an effective weight loss agent, prevented diabetes in obese-prone rats by reducing lipid accumulation. (65)

Omega-3 free fatty acids and niacin had a positive lowering effect on the hyperlipidemia of T2D. (66)

Intake of magnesium-rich foods had a beneficial effect on the lipid profile in diabetic patients with no significant effect on blood glucose levels. (67)

The sulfa compounds in onions (*Allium cepa*) were effective in lowering plasma glucose concentrations and body weight in experimental diabetic rats. (68) In addition to its antioxidative and anti-inflammatory properties, garlic (*Allium sativum*) acted as an insulin secretagogue and sensitizer in preventing diabetes progression and related complications. (69) Dietary intake of minimally refined cereal fiber grain was associated with reduced risk of diabetes in women. (70) Similarly, beans, lentils, and seeds reduced the blood glucose concentration when compared to whole meal breads and dairy fat. (71)

Chromium picolinate has been shown to optimize insulin function and reduce hyperglycemia and hyperinsulinemia in clinical trials. (72) Despite the untoward health effects of high intake of coffee (particularly on the cardiovascular system), the presence of some ingredients (chlorogenic acid, lignans, and quinides) reduced glucose uptake and inhibit oxidative stress and inflammation. (73) A dietary pattern with higher intake of soy products reduced the risk of type 2 diabetes in the Singapore Chinese Health Study. (74) An aqueous extract of *Cucumis trigonis* (cucumber) had beneficial effects in reducing elevated blood glucose level and lipid profile in diabetic rats. (75)

Vitamin E (tocopherols) improved insulin sensitivity through enhanced adiponectin expression. (76) Vitamin C supplementation restored T-cell function in diabetic rats. (77) The flavonoid, quercetin, exerted DNA-antioxidative protective effects on the liver, kidney, and immune systems of diabetic mice. It is found in high contents in apples. (78)

In epidemiological studies, vitamin D deficiency was found to be linked to the onset of type 2 diabetes through loss of vascular protection and immunomodulatory effects. (79) DHEA injections improved hyperglycemia and increased glucose uptake and utilization in skeletal muscle in streptozotocin-induced diabetic rats. (80)

Most of these studies have been done on experimental animals. Though a paradigm shift is needed to accept logical outcomes in the absence of hard evidence, in our present medical climate, human clinical trials are demanded by a majority of researchers and clinical practitioners in order for the results to be accepted as evidence-based fact.

Caution: High intakes of omega-3 fish oil (but not plant-based omega-3 fatty acids) were associated with increased risk for type 2 diabetes. (81)

**Botanical supplementation for diabetes mellitus is prevalent worldwide.

Cinnamon	Astragalus	Green tea	Bitter melon
Insulina leaf	Dandelion leaf	Nettles	Psyllium
Gymnestra sylvestre	Fenugreek	Eucalyptus	Papaya
Aloe vera	Lemongrass	Gooseberry leaf	Prickly pear cactus

Table 2: Botanicals Beneficial to Type 2 Diabetes Mellitus.

In a human clinical trial, cinnamon (*Cinnamomi cassiae*) intake of 2 g per day for twelve weeks significantly reduced the HbA1c among poorly controlled type 2 diabetic patients by increasing insulin sensitivity and reducing serum and hepatic lipids. (82) Astragalus polysaccharides were effective in the prevention of type 1 diabetes by correcting the imbalance between Th1/Th2 cytokines. (83) Green tea catechins lowered the hemoglobin A1c level in individuals with borderline diabetes when taken daily. (84)

Bitter melon (*Mormordica charantia*), also known as maidenapple and bitter gourd, improved insulin sensitivity and insulin signaling by increasing skeletal muscle tyrosine phosphorylation in diabetic rats. (85) An aqueous extract from insulina leaf (*Cissus sicyoides)* showed hypoglycemic and anti-lipemic effects in the treatment of alloxan-induced type 2 diabetes mellitus in rats. (86) Extracts of dandelion leaf (*Taraxacum officinale*) and stinging nettle (*Urtica dioica*) lowered blood glucose through their inhibitory activity on the enzyme, alpha-glucosidase. (87) The addition of psyllium husk fiber to the diets of men with T2D improved glycemic and lipid control. (88) *Gymnestra sylvestre* (gumar) is an ayurvedic herbal widely used in Asia for its hypoglycemic activity. Hepatotoxicity with overuse has recently been reported as a serious adverse effect. (89) Fenugreek seed powder (*Trigonella foenum-gracum*) showed hypoglycemic, hypolipidemic and immunomodulatory properties in diabetic/obese patients and in those under chemotherapeutic interventions. (90) Eucalyptus leaves *(E. globulus*) partially restored pancreatic beta cells and repaired STZ-induced damage to diabetic rats in a dose-dependent manner. (91) A fermented preparation of *Carica papaya* was used to reduce the effects of oxidative stress and stabilized diabetes in patients with severe blood dyscrasias. (92) Emodin, a biologically active compound in *Aloe vera,* appeared to have a significant hypoglycemic effect by regulating carbohydrate metabolizing enzymes. (93) The *Cymbopogon proximus* variety of lemongrass significantly reduced elevated blood glucose in alloxan-induced diabetic rats by its regulation on the hepatic activity of the cytochrome P450 system. (94) Gooseberry leaf (*Emblica officinalis*) or *aamla*, reduce oxidative stress in STZ-induced diabetic rats. (95) Prickly pear cactus (*Opuntia dellinii*) exerted its hypoglycemic effect by protecting the liver from peroxidation damage and improving the sensitivity and response of target cells to insulin in diabetic mice. (96)

Additional botanicals used in traditional medicine to treat diabetes are: *Antigonon leptopus, Bidens pilosa, Bidens alba, Bixa orellana, Bontia daphnoides, Catharanthus roseus, Cocos nucifera, Gomphrena globosa, Laportea aestuans, Morus alba, Phyllanthus urinaria, Spiranthes acaulis* (97) and *Jambolan* and *Pterocarpus marsupium.*

Exercise improves insulin resistance in both smooth and skeletal muscles, and glucose uptake at the cellular level. Active muscles can extract glucose from the blood more efficiently than resting muscle for energy conversion. Poor circulation from inactivity leads to oxygen deprivation in all cells. A good thirty to forty-minute walk at least three times a week is good for circulation and helps to lower blood sugar. (98)

(See Chapter Seven: Exercise and Eye Health)

Case Scenario Four: A 63-year-old female had a sudden decrease in vision due to a vitreous hemorrhage. She has a history of insulin-dependent diabetes for the past fifteen years and has had previous focal and panretinal laser treatments. In addition to conventional treatment, what else can be suggested to reduce active bleeding in the posterior chamber?

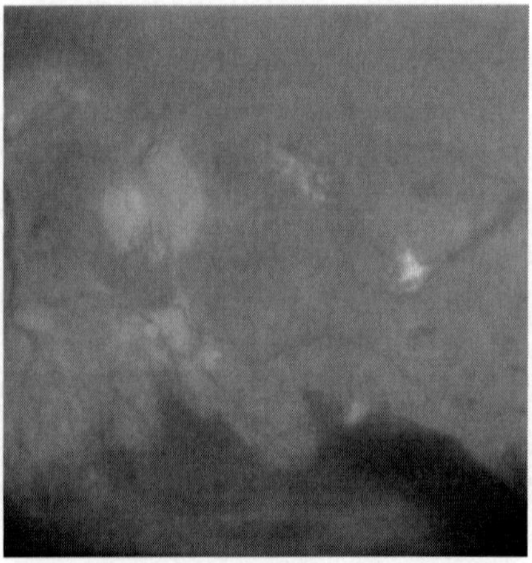

diabetic vitreo-retinal hemorrhage

It is prudent and practical to get a history of anticoagulant, herbal, and supplement use. Compounds that should be avoided or discontinued due to their blood thinning properties are: *Ginkgo biloba*, garlic, ginger, ginseng, glucosamine chondroitin, grapefruit juice, vitamin E, echinacea, feverfew, fenugreek, omega-3 fish oil, flaxseed oil, danshen, cayenne pepper, dong quai, devil's claw, turkey tail, turmeric, licorice, reischii, coenzyme Q10, bilberry, NSAIDs, and aspirin.

Case Scenario Five: A 50-year-old female presents with BCVA 20/25 and an essentially normal exam. She gives a family history of a parent and an aunt who are blind from macular degeneration. She is overweight, eats fast-food five times a week and has a pack-a-day cigarette habit. She asks, "What can I do to prevent macular degeneration?"

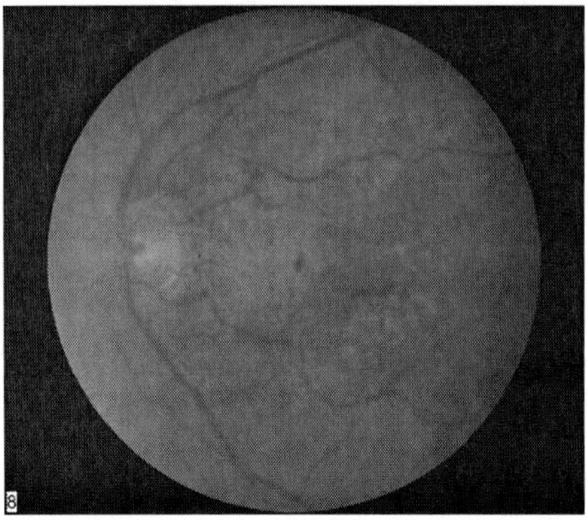

age-related macular degeneration

Age-related macular degeneration (ARMD) is a leading cause of blindness in individuals over the age of sixty. It is a degenerative condition of the macula, characterized by the dysfunction and eventual death of the retinal photoreceptors. Risk factors include aging, cigarette smoking, genetic predisposition, presence of drusen, deficiency of antioxidant levels, excessive exposure to UV radiation and toxins, reduced kidney function, and hypertension. (99) Pathology is characterized by reduction in levels of the macular pigments, lutein, and zeaxanthin, which function as blue-light filters and antioxidants, retinal anoxia, retinal pigment epithelium atrophy, poor retinal circulation, and oxidative stress. The AREDS study shows that the consumption of whole foods or supplements that contain lutein and zeaxanthin increases macular pigment density and has the potential to preserve vision and prevent or slow further degeneration. (100) Observational studies suggested a benefit from increased intake of dietary macular xanthophylls and minerals zinc and copper. (101) (102) (103) Evidence for the benefits of the use of omega-3 fatty acids for a.m. treatment and prevention exists in some circles and remains controversial in others.(104) (105)

Consuming diets that provide low dietary glycemic index intakes of vitamin C and E, lutein/zeaxanthin, DHA and EPA from AREDS baseline information, were associated with the greatest reduction in risk for prevalent drusen and advanced AMD. (106)

Taking preventive measures against developing age-related macular degeneration, especially for those with risk factors, makes good sense.

Recommendations for Complementary Prevention and Treatment of Age-Related Macular Degeneration (ARMD) in Medium to High-Risk Individuals:

1. Stop smoking (107)
2. Use protection from excessive UV radiation (wraparound sunglasses with UV 400 filter)(108)
3. Avoid excessive intake of antihistamines, diuretics, decongestants, beta-blockers, narcotics, antimetabolite cancer drugs, and saturated fats (proinflammatory)
4. Consume whole foods and/or antioxidant supplements with lutein (2-10mg), zeaxanthin, omega-3 fatty acids (1000 mg), and berry extracts (anti-inflammatory)
5. Glutathione (in cruciferous vegetables like onions, garlic, asparagus) (109)
6. Minerals: Zinc, chromium, copper, and magnesium
7. Melatonin 3 mg qhs
8. Botanicals: Turmeric 400–500 mg
9. Chelation therapy in cases of toxicity

Hydroquinone is a major proinflammatory oxidant in cigarette smoke, which was found to induce actin rearrangement and membrane bleb formation in RPE cells and sub-RPE deposits in mice. (110)

Melatonin has receptors located in the RPE, which act as neuromodulators to stimulate telomerase activity. A clinical trial showed that 3 mg given at bedtime for three months to a.m. patients reduced pathologic macular changes. (111)

Curcumin, the active ingredient in turmeric (*Curcuma longa*), protected retinal cells from oxidant and light-stress-induced cell death by inhibiting the NF-kB enzyme activation and down-regulation of cellular inflammatory genes. (112)

Green tea catechins and grape resveratrol have the potential to reduce macular degeneration through their ability to ameliorate ocular oxidative stress. However, the only proven effective preventive measures are stopping smoking and the AREDS formula of lutein, zeaxanthin, omega-3, and berry extracts.

Lut/Zea	**Omega-3**	**Vitamin C**	**Copper**	**Zinc**
Green leafy vegetables	Cold water fish (salmon, tuna,)	Citrus fruit	Shellfish	Turkey (dark meat)
Blueberries	Soy products	Acerolas	Grains	Oysters
Grapes	Yogurt	Mango	Beans	Pumpkin seeds
Melons	Flaxseed	Guava	Organ meats	Milk
Bilberry	Olive oil	Kiwi	Dried fruit	Nuts

Table 3: Antioxidant-Rich Foods for Macular Degeneration:

In the Beaver Dam eye study, though an association was found between beer consumption, retinal drusen in men, and exudative macular degeneration, and an inverse relationship was found between moderate wine intake and ARMD, the overall consumption of alcoholic beverages was not found to be an important risk factor for the incidence of ARMD. Resveratrol, a component in wine, has shown some cytoprotective effects and prevention of VEGF secretion which may be of benefit in a.m. treatment. (113) (114) (115)

The Task Force on Complementary Therapies found no strong scientific evidence for the effectiveness of microcurrent stimulation in the treatment of age-related macular degeneration.

(See Acupuncture as an effective treatment for certain stages of macular degeneration in Chapter Ten)

References for Chapter Four:

1. Christen WG, et al. Age-related cataract in a randomized trial of vitamins E and C in men. Arch Ophthalmol. 2010 Nov; 128(11):1397-405.
2. Seddon JM. Multivitamin-multimineral supplements and eye disease: age-related macular degeneration and cataract. Am J Clin Nutr. 2007 Jan; 85(1):304S-307S.
3. Delcourt C, et al. Risk factors for cortical, nuclear, and posterior subcapsular cataracts: the POLA study. Pathologies Oculaires Liées à l'Age. Am J Epidemiol. 2000 Mar 1; 151(5):497-504.
4. Obara Y. [The oxidative stress in the cataract formation]. Nippon Ganka Gakkai Zasshi. 1995 Dec; 99(12): 1303-41.
5. Zhang M, et al. Topical metal chelation therapy ameliorates oxidation-induced toxicity in diabetic cataract. J Toxicol Environ Health A. 2011 Jan; 74(6):380-91.
6. Hodge WG, Witcher JP, Satariano W.Risk factors for age-related cataracts. Epidemiol Rev. 1995; 17(2):336-46.
7. Anduze, AL. Ultraviolet radiation and cataract development in the U.S. Virgin Islands. J Cataract Refract Surg. Mar 1993. Vol.19; 298-300.
8. Aman K, et al. Effect of high-glucose levels on protein oxidation in cultured lens cells, and in crystalline and albumin solution and its inhibition by vitamin B6 and N-acetylcysteine: its possible relevance to cataract formation in diabetes. Free Radical Biology and Medicine. Vol 33, Issue 12, Dec 15, 2002; 1615-21.
9. James ER.The etiology of steroid cataract. J Ocul Pharmacol Ther.; 23(5): 403-20.
10. Bair B, et al. Cataracts in atopic Dermatitis: A Case Presentation and Review of the Literature. Arch Dermatol. 2011 Jan 17.
11. Shichi H. Cataract formation and prevention. Expert Opin Investig Drugs.; 13(6):691-701.
12. Babizhayev MA, et al. N-Acetylcarnosine sustained drug delivery eyedrops to control the signs of ageless vision… Clin Interv Aging. 2009;4: 31-50.

13. Babizhayev MA, et al. N-acetylcarnosine lubricant eyedrops possess all-in-one universal antioxidant protective effects of L-carnosine in aqueous and lipid membrane environments,aldehyde scavenging, and transglycation activities inherent to cataracts: a clinical study… Am J ther. 2009 Nov-Dec; 16(6):517-33.
14. Akiyama N, et al. 5-S-GAD. A novel radical scavenging compound, prevents lens opacity development. Free Radical Biol Med. 2009 Feb 15; 46(4): 511-9
15. Baraldi P, et al. Medical treatment of senile cataract: Clinical investigation of bendazac-lysine using objective and subjective methods. Graefe's Archive for Clinical and Experimental Ophthalmology. Vol.228, No.2, 105-111.
16. Anitha TS, et al. Prevention of Selenite-Induced Cataractogenesis by an Ethanolic Extract of Cineraria maritime: An Experimental Evaluation of the Traditional Eye Medication. Biol Trace Elem Res. 2010 Oct 15.
17. Bingel U, Colloca L, Vase L. Mechanisms and Clinical Implications of the Placebo Effect: Is There a Potential for the Elderly? A Mini-Review.Gerontology. 2010 Oct 21.
18. Pollo A, Benedetti F. The placebo response: neurobiological and clinical issues of neurological relevance. Prog Brain Res.2009; 175:283-94.
19. Babizhayev MA. New concept in nutrition for the maintenance of the aging eye redox regulation and therapeutic treatment of cataract disease; synergism of natural antioxidant imidazole-containing amino acid-based compounds, chaperone, and glutathione boosting agents:a systemic perspective on aging and longevity emerged from studies in humans. Am J Ther.2010 Jul-Aug;17(4):373-89.
20. Sheck L, Davies J, Wilson G. Selenium and ocular health in New Zealand. N Z Med J. 2010 Jun 11; 123(1316): 85-94.
21. Meyer LM, et al. Absence of glutaredoxin1 increases lens susceptibility to oxidative stress induced by UVR-B. Exp Eye Res. 2009 Dec; 89(6):833-9.

22. Yao K, et al. Epigallocatechin gallate protects against oxidative stress-induced mitochondria- dependent apoptosis in human lens epithelial cells. Mol Vis. 2008 Jan 31; 14:217-23.
23. Manikandan R, et al. Curcumin prevents free radical-mediated cataractogenesis through modulations in lens calcium.Free Radic Biol Med. 2010 Feb 15; 48(4): 483-92.
24. Karunakaran-Datt A, Kennepohl P. Redox photochemistry of methionine by sulfur K-edge X-ray Absorption spectroscopy: potential implications for cataract formation. J Am Chem Soc. 2009 Mar 18; 131(10):3577-82.
25. Leske MC, et al. Centrum Use and Progression of Age-Related Cataract in the Age-Related Eye Disease Study. A Propensity Score Approach. AREDS Report No. 21. And Antioxidant Vitamins and Nuclear Opacities. The Longitudinal Cataract Study. Ophthalmol 2006; 113:1264-70.
26. Mosad SM, et al. Lens cadmium, lead, and serum vitamins C,E, and beta carotene in cataractous smoking patients. Curr Eye Res. 2010 Jan; 35(1):23-30.
27. Agarwal R, et al. Current concepts in pathophysiology of glaucoma. Indian J Ophthalmol. 2009 Jul-Aug; 57(4):257-66.
28. Ray K, Mookherjee S. Molecular complexity of primary open angle glaucoma: current concepts. J Genet. 2009 Dec; 88(4): 451-67.
29. Leske MC, et al. Risk factors for incident open-angle glaucoma: the Barbados Eye Studies. Ophthalmology. 2008 Jan; 115(1):85-93.
30. He Z, Vingrys AJ, Armitage JA, Bui BV. The role of blood pressure inglaucoma. Clin Exp Optom. 2011 Jan 24. (Epub ahead of print)
31. Neroev VV, Zueva MV, Kalamkarov GR. [Molecular mechanisms in retinal ischemia]. Vestn Oftalmol. 2010 May-Jun; 126(3):59-64.
32. Medeiros FA, et al. The relationship between intraocular pressure and progressive retinal nerve fiber layer loss in glaucoma. Ophthalmology. 2009 Jun; 116(6):1125-33.
33. Tataru LC, Bogdanici CM. [Glaucoma—neurodegenerative disease]. Rev Med Chir Soc Med Nat Iasi. 2009 Oct-Dec; 113(4):1120-5.

34. Istrate B. [Immunological aspects in glaucoma]. Oftalmologia. 2010;54(2):44-7
35. Turgut B, et al Levels of circulating homocysteine, vitamin B6, vitamin B12, and folate in different types of open-angle glaucoma. Clin Interv Aging. 2010Apr 26; 5:133-9.
36. Parikh RS, Parikh SR.Alternative therapy in glaucoma management: is there any role? Indian J Ophthalmol. 2011 Jan; 59 Suppl:S 158-60.
37. Ritch R. Potential role for Gingko biloba extract in the treatment of glaucoma. Med Hypotheses. 2000 Feb; 54(2):221-35.
38. Chung HS, et al. Gingko biloba extract increases ocular blood flow velocity. J Ocul Pharmacol Ther. 1999 Jun; 15(3):233-40.
39. Quaranta L, et al. Effect of Gingko biloba extract on preexisting visual field damage in normal tension glaucoma. Ophthalmology. 2003 Feb; 110(2):359-62.
40. Russo R, et al. Rational basis for the development of coenzyme Q10 as a neurotherapeutic agent for retinal protection. Prog Brain Res. 2008; 173: 575-82.
41. Yuki K, et al. Reduced-serum vitamin C and increased uric acid levels in normal-tension glaucoma. Graefes Arch Clin Exp Ophthalmol. 2010 Feb; 248(2):243-8.
42. Bruhn RL, et al. Relationship between glaucoma and selenium levels in plasma and aqueous humour. Br J Ophthalmol. 2009 Sep; 93(9):1155-8.
43. Kang JH, et al. Dietary fat consumption and primary open-angle glaucoma. Am J Clin Nutr. 2004 May;79(5):755-64.
44. Nguyen CT, et al. Dietary omega-3 fatty acids decrease intraocular pressure with age by increasing aqueous outflow. Invest Ophthalmol Vis Sci. 2007 Feb; 48(2):756-62.
45. Miyamoto N, et al. Quercetin Induces the Expression of Peroxiredoxins 3 and 5 via the Nrf/NRF1 Transcription Pathway. Invest Ophthalmol Vis Sci. 2011 Feb 22; 52(2):1055-63.
46. Mozaffarieh M, et al. The potential value of natural antioxidative treatment in glaucoma. Surv Ophthalmol. 2008 Sep-Oct; 53(5):479-505.

47. Bagchi D, et al. Anti-angiogenic, antioxidant, and anti-carcinogenic properties of a novel anthocyanin-rich berry extract formula. Biochemistry (Mosc). 2004 Jan; 69(1):75-80.
48. Merritt JC, et al. Effect of Marijuana on Intraocular and Blood Pressure in Glaucoma. Ophthalmol. 1980 Mar; 87(3): 222-8
49. Green K. Marijuana smoking vs cannabinoids for glaucoma therapy. Arch Ophthalmol. 1998 Nov; 116(11):1433-7.
50. Merritt JC, et al.Topical delta 9-tetrahydrocannabinol in hypertensive glaucomas. J. Pharmacol. 1981 Jan; 33(1):40-1
51. Merritt JC. Glaucoma, hypertension, and marijuana. J Natl Med Assoc. 1982 Aug; 74(8):715-6.
52. Merritt JC, et al.Topical delta 9-tetrahydrocannabinol and aqueous dynamics in glaucoma. J Clin Pharacol. 1981 Aug-Sep; 21(8-9 Suppl):467S-471S.
53. Risner D, et al.Effects of exercise on intraocular pressure and ocular blood flow: a review. J Glaucoma. 2009 Aug; 18(6):429-36.
54 Passo MS, et al. Exercise training reduces intraocular pressure among subjects suspected of having glaucoma. Arch Ophthalmol. 1991 Aug; 109(8):1096-8.
55. Ray S, Mehra KS, Misra S, Singh R. Plasma cortisol in glaucoma. Ann Ophthalmol. 1977 Sep; 9(9):1151-4.
56. Weitzman ED, et al. Correlative 24-hour relationship between intraocular pressure and plasma cortisol in normal subjects and patients with glaucoma. Br J Ophthalmol. 1975 Oct; 59(10):566-72.
57. Head KA. Natural therapies for ocular disorders, part two: cataracts and glaucoma. Altern Med rev. 2001 Apr; 6(2):141-66.
58. Golbidi S, Ebadi SA, Laher I. Antioxidants in the Treatment of diabetes. Curr Diabetes Rev. 2011 Feb 7.
59. Lee T, Dugoua JJ. Nutritional Supplements and Their Effect on Glucose Control. Curr Diab Rep. 2011 Feb 8.
60. Mohammad G, Kowluru RA. Novel Role of Mitochondrial Matrix Metalloproteinase-2 in the Development of Diabetic Retinopathy. Invest Ophthalmol Vis Sci. 2011 Feb 23.

61. Ergul A. Endothelin-1 and diabetic complications: Focus on the vasculature. Pharmacol Res. 2011 Feb 1.
62. Esposito K, Giugliano D. Increased consumption of green leafy vegetables, but not fruit, vegetables or fruit and vegetables combined, is associated with reduced incidence of type 2 diabetes. Evid Based Med. 2011 Feb; 16(1):27-8.
63. Sargent LA, et al. Fruit and vegetable intake and population glycolated haemoglobin levels: the EPIC-Norfolk Study. Eur J Clin Nutr. 2001 May; 55(5):342-8.
64. Serpeloni JM, et al. Lutein improves antioxidant defense in vivo and protects against DNA damage and chromosome instability induced by cisplatin. Arch Toxicol. 2010 Oct; 84(10):811-22.
65. Song KH, et al. alpha-Lipoic acid prevents diabetes mellitus in diabetes-prone obese rats. Biochem Biophys Res Commun. 2005 Jan 7; 326(1):197-202.
66. Vergès B. Combination lipid therapy in type 2 diabetes mellitus. Expert Opin Pharmacother. 2011 Feb 16.
67. Lal J, et al. Effect of oral magnesium supplementation on the lipid profile and blood glucose of patients with type 2 diabetes mellitus. J Assoc Physicians India. 2003 Jan; 51:37-42.
68. Kook S, Kim GH, Choi K.The antidiabetic effect of onion and garlic in experimental diabetic rats: meta-analysis. J Med Food. 2009 Jun; 12(3):552-60.
69. Liu CT, Sheen LY, Lii CK.Does garlic have a role as an antidiabetic agent?. Mol Nutr Food Res. 2007 Nov; 51(11):1353-64.
70. Salmerón J, et al. Dietary fiber, glycemic load, and risk of non-insulin-dependent diabetes mellitus in women. JAMA. 1997 Feb 12; 277(6):472-7.
71. Jenkins DJ, et al. Effect of guar crispbread with cereal products and leguminous seeds on blood glucose concentrations of diabetics. Br Med J. 1980 Nov 8; 281(6250):1248-50.
72. Broadhurst CL, Domenico P. Clinical studies on chromium picolinate supplementation in diabetes mellitus—a review. Diabetes Technol Ther. 2006 Dec; 8(6):677-87.
73. Kempf K, Martin S. [Coffee and diabetes]. Med Klin (Munich). 2010 Dec; 105(12):910-5.

74. Odegaard AO, et al. Dietary Patterns and Incident Type 2 Diabetes in Chinese men and women: The Singapore Chinese Health Study. Diabetes Care. 2011 Feb 17.
75. Antidiabetic activity of aqueous fruit extract of Cucumis trigonis Roxb. in streptozotocin-induced-diabetic rats. Salahuddin M, et al. J Ethnopharmacol. 2010 Feb 3; 127(2):565-7.
76. Gray B, Swick J, Ronnenberg AG. Vitamin E and adiponectin: proposed mechanism for vitamin E induced improvement in insulin sensitivity. Nutr Rev. 2011 Mar; 69(3):155-61.
77. Badr G, et al. Vitamin C supplementation reconstitutes polyfunctional T cells in streptozotocin-induced diabetic rats. Eur J Nutr. 2011 Feb 25.
78. Orsolic N, et al. DNA-protective effects of quercetin or naringenin in alloxan-induced diabetic mice. Eur J Pharmacol. 2011 Jan 28.
79. Devaraj S, et al.Low vitamin d levels correlate with the proinflammatory state in type 1 diabetic subjects with and without microvascular complications. Am J Clin Pathol. 2011 Mar; 135(3):429-33.
80. Sato K, et al. DHEA improves impaired activation of Akt and PKC zeta/lambda-GLUT4 pathway in skeletal muscle and improves hyperglycaemia in streptozotocin-induced diabetes rats. Acta Physiol oxf. 2009 Nov; 197(3):217-25.
81. Djoussé L, et al. Dietary omega-3 fatty acids and fish consumption and risk of type 2 diabetes. Am J Clin Nutr. 2011 Jan; 93(1):143-50.
82. Aikilen R, et al. Glycated haemoglobin and blood pressure-lowering effect of cinnamon in multi-ethnic Type 2 diabetic patients in the UK: a randomized, placebo-controlled, double-blind clinical trial. Diabet Med. 2010 Oct; 27(10):1159-67.
83. Chen W, et al. Astragalus polysaccharides:an effective treatment for diabetes prevention in NOD mice. Exp Clin Endocrinol Diabetes. 2008 Aug; 116(8):468-74.
84. Fukino Y, et al. Randomized controlled trial for an effect of green tea-extract powder supplementation on glucose abnormalities. Eur J Clin Nutr. 2008 Aug; 62(8): 953-60.
85. Sridhar MG, et al. Bitter gourd (Mormordica charantia) improves insulin sensitivity by increasing skeletal muscle insulin-stimulated

IRS-1 tyrosine phosphorylation in high-fat-fed rats. Br J Nutr. 2008 Apr 99(4): 806-12.

86. Viana GS, et al. Hypoglycemic and anti-lipemic effects of the aqueous extract from Cissus sicyoides. BMC Pharmacol. 2004 Jun 8; 4: 9.
87. Onal S, et al. Inhibition of alpha-glucosidase by aqueous extracts of some potent antidiabetic medicinal herbs. Prep Biochem Biotechnol. 2005; 35(1):29-36.
88. Anderson JW et al. Effects of psyllium on glucose & serum lipid responses in men with type 2 diabetes & hypercholesterolemia. Am J Clin Nutr.1999 Oct; 70(4):466-73.
89. Shiyovich A, et al. Toxic hepatitis induced by Gymnema sylvestre, a natural remedy for type 2 diabetes mellitus. Am J Med Sci. 2010 Dec; 340(6): 514-7.
90. Ramadan G, El-Beih NM, Abd el-Kareem HF. Anti-metabolic syndrome and immunostimulant activities of Egyptian fenugreek seeds in diabetic/obese and immunosuppressive rat modelsBr J Nutr. 2010 Dec 23:1-10.
91. Mahmoudzadeh-Sagheb H, et al. Antidiabetic effects of Eucalyptus globulus on pancreatic islets: a stereological study. Folia Morphol (Warsz). 2010 May; 69(2):112-8.
92. Amer J, et al. Fermented papaya preparation as redox regulator in blood cells of beta-thalassemic mice and patients. Phytother res. 2008 Jun;22(6):820-8
93. Rajasekaran S, et al. Hypoglycemic effect of Aloe vera gel on streptozotocin-induced diabetes in experimental ratsJ Med Food. 2004 Spring; 7(1):61-6.
94. Sheweita SA, et al. Effect of some hypoglycemic herbs on the activity of phase I and II drug-metabolizing enzymes in alloxan-induced diabetis rats. Toxicology. 2002 May 24; 174(2):131-9.
95. Yokozawa T, et al. Amla (Emplica officinalis Gaertn.) prevents dyslipidaemia and oxidative stress in the ageing process. Br J Nutr. 2007 Jun; 97(6):1187-95.
96. Zhao LY, et al. Antidiabetic effect of a newly identified component of Opuntia dillenii polysaccharides. Phytomedicine. 2011 Feb 5.

97. Lans CA. Ethnomedicines used in Trinidad and Tobago for urinary problems and diabetes mellitus. J Ethnobiol Ethnomed. 2006 Oct 13; 2:45.
98. Malaysz T, et al. Beneficial effects of treadmill training in experimental diabetic nerve regeneration. Clinics (Sao Paolo). 2010; 65(12):1329-37.
99. Tomany SC, et al. Risk factors for incident age-related macular degeneration: pooled findings from 3 continents. Ophthalmology. 2004 Jul; 111(7):1280-7.
100. Carpentier S, Knaus M, Suh M. Associations between lutein, zeaxanthin, and age-related macular degeneration: an overview. Crit Rev Food Sci Nutr. 2009 Apr; 49(4):313-26.
101. Wong IY, Koo SC, Chan CW.Prevention of age-related macular degeneration. Int Ophthalmol. 2011 Feb; 31(1):73-82.
102. Krishnadev N, Meleth AD, Chew EY. Nutritional supplements for age-related macular degeneration. Curr Opin Ophthalmol. 2010 May; 21(3):184-9
103. Rehak M, Fric E, Wiedermann P. [Lutein and antioxidants in the prevention of age-related macular degeneration]. Ophthalmologe. 2008 Jan; 105(1):37-8.
104. Chong EW, et al. Dietary omega-3 fatty acid and fish intake in the primary prevention of age-related macular degeneration: a systemic review and meta- analysis. Arch Ophthalmol. 2008 Jun; 126(6):826-33.
105. Hodge WG, et al.Evidence for effect of omega-3 fatty acids on progression of age-related macular degeneration: a systemic review. Retina. 2007 Feb; 27(2):216-21.
106. Chiu CJ, et al. Dietary compound score and risk of age-related macular degeneration in the age-related eye disease study. Ophthalmology. 2009 May; 116(5):939-46.
107. Seddon JM, George S, Rosner B. Seddon JM, George S, Rosner B. Cigarette smoking, fish consumption, omega-3 fatty acid intake and associations with age-related macular degeneration: the US Twin Study of Age-Related Macular Degeneration. Arch Ophthalmol. 2006 Jul; 124(7):995-1001.

108. Marc RE, et al. Extreme retinal remodeling triggered by light damage: imply-cations for age related macular degeneration. Mol Vis. 2008 Apr 25; 14:782-806.
109. Guven M, et al. Glutathione S-Transferase M1, GSTT1 and GSTP1 Genetic Polymorphisms and the Risk of Age-Related Macular Degeneration. Ophthalmic Res. 2011 Jan5; 46(1)31:31-37.
110. Pons M, et al. Cigarette smoke-related hydroquinone induces filamentous actin reorganization and heat shock protein 27 phosphorylation through p38 and extraocular signal-regulated kinase ½ in retinal pigment epithelium: implications for age-related macular degeneration. Am J Pathol. 2010 Sep; 177(3):1198-213.
111. Rasmanesh R. Potential of melatonin to treat or prevent age-related macular degeneration through stimulation of telomerase activity. Med Hypotheses. 2010 Sep 28.
112. Mandal MN, et al. Curcumin protects retinal cells from light-and oxidant stress-induced cell death. Free Radic Biol Med. 2009 Mar 1; 46(5):672-9.
113. Moss SE, Klein R, Klein BE, et al. Alcohol consumption and the 5-year incidence of age-related maculopathy: the Beaver Dam eye study. Ophthalmology 1998 May; 105(5):789-94.
114. Alcohol use and age-related maculopathy in the Beaver Dam eye study. Am J Ophthalmol. 1995 Aug: 120(2): 190-6.
115. Dugas B.et al.Effects of oxysterols on cell viability, inflammatory cytokines, VEGF, and reactive oxygen species production on human retinal cells: cytoprotective effects and prevention of VEGF secretion by resveratrol. Eur J Nutr.2010 Oct; 49(7):435-46.

Nutrition and the Eye

The systemic factors that influence the onset and progression of disease include alterations in the cardiovascular system, central, and autonomic nervous systems, endocrine, and immune systems as well as other physical and psychological processes. (1) Contributing factors to the onset and progression of glaucoma, cataracts, diabetic retinopathy, macular degeneration, neurodegenerative, and autoimmune diseases are as follows: Oxidative stress, free radical damage, inflammation, toxicity effects, declined immune defenses, decreased circulation, and basic dehydration. Responses to the medical and surgical treatment and ultimately the health of the eyes is reflective to the medical status of the body and mind; that which can neutralize or correct the causes of eye disease can also improve or slow the progression of the malady.

Good nutrition is essential to the healthy maintenance of all organ systems. Whole food is better, safer and more effective than supplements.

Case Scenario One: A 54-year-old patient wishes to have discussion on which foods and supplements are best for vision? She asks, "Why should I take them? Do they really work? How and when should I take them? What are the best ones to take? What are the side effects?"

First, the focus of the examination should be on the patient and not on the nutritional products in question. The doctor should listen attentively, respect, and address the patients' concerns. Second, he or she should make proper use of communication and teaching skills when concerned with practical protocols of diet and lifestyle behaviors that support the eye in order to impart logical and truthful information. Although patients are well aware of the availability, benefits, and intended actions of foods and supplements, they still want the doctor's opinion and the value of his or her suggestive influence.

Why? Making good food choices in all cases and taking supplements when indicated make good_scientific sense. It may be beneficial to take supplements when in situations where good quality whole food is unavailable, such as when travelling.

In life, we utilize food (burn fuel), which provides energy and releases free radicals. The latter interact with body cells to retrieve a lost electron. In the process of retrieval, free radicals cause changes in physiology, which leads to the destruction of lipids, proteins and DNA, resulting in cell necrosis and death. The ability of antioxidants to inhibit, neutralize, or stimulate enzymes to repair damage provides a protective effect on cells, tissues, and organs. (2) (3)Most patients will understand and accept the concept regarding the benefits of antioxidants, but some doctors are still skeptical and demand hard evidence of such conclusions._There is ample evidence to support that taking antioxidant supplements such as lutein, zeaxanthin, and zinc (AREDS II) is beneficial as well as increasing dietary intake of omega-3 fatty acids for individuals at high risk for age-related macular degeneration. (4) (5)

While low levels of antioxidants are associated with many disease processes, taking supplements alone is not mandatory for good health nor will it completely restore damaged organs.

Better experimental designs are needed to identify the intake dosage using whole foods, plasma concentrations, and rate of risk of particular diseases. Beware of studies done by pharmaceutical companies as these can be biased and skewed in whatever direction desired and give rise to under or over reporting of negative or positive results. Likewise, beware of studies that imply that supplements are the magic bullet to recovery or prevention of disease.

Evidence-based studies use the results of clinical expertise and research to support the premise that intervention improves outcomes. Experimental evidence is based on laboratory models which are then applied to clinical reality. However, studies involving large cohorts of human individuals are not always uniform in that they have different starting points and different departures in behavior. Not all the cataracts in a group will be at exactly the same stage or be of the same type, and certainly they will not all be at the same level of health. Skeptics should refer to the results of evidence-based studies from the National Institutes of Health (NIH), the Dietary Supplement Health and Education Act (DSHEA) of 1994, and the AREDS I and II studies. (6) (7) (8)

The quality of our food supply is inadequate to provide natural therapeutic agents in optimal dosages. The trend toward local, organic produce is real, but remains small in scale and does not reach the majority of the population. Though more physicians and policy makers are changing their stance to support the facts that nutritional supplements and vitamins do in fact play a key role in the prevention of many chronic diseases, like cancer, depression, heart disease, osteoporosis, and eye disease, the impact of change has not yet been felt. Patients are using supplements, and those who may be using them incorrectly need to be informed. Not recommending or not discussing their use may cause greater harm.

Much of health care revolves around cost effectiveness. Note that the cost of anti-VEGF injections for a.m. far outstrips the cost of preventive supplementation.

Yet research is directed toward crisis management instead of prevention.

Integrative medicine compliments conventional medicine. It is not competitive nor is it intended as a replacement. Its purpose is to provide information that will support good health.

Coldwater fish (Omega-3)	Green leafy vegetables	Root vegetables	Fruit, yellow vegetables	Extra virgin olive oil
Eggs	Soy	Red wine	Berries	Nuts and seeds

Table 1: Best Foods for Healthy Eyes:

How do they work in the prevention of macular degeneration?

Salmon, sardines, tuna, cod and mackerel, olive oil, nuts and seeds, cereal grains, and pasta, are all good sources of omega-3 fatty acids, decosahexaenoic acid (DHA), and eicosapentaenoic acid (EPA), which may slow the progression of vision loss from age-related macular degeneration and reverse the signs of dry eye syndrome. These polyunsaturated fats are good for RPE protection, and free radical neutralization, and they keep lupofuscin accumulation in check. (9) (10) Patients with low linoleic acid levels had a higher incidence of ARMD. (11) Note that the Beaver Dam, Blue Mountain, Framingham, American Journal of Clinical Nutrition, AREDS I and II studies all showed a positive correlation of the preventive effects of omega-3 fatty acids on ARMD. The ability of omega-3 oils to neutralize or prevent the accumulation of low-density lipoproteins in the retina after active remodeling within the RPE may be part of the mechanism of action. (12) Since inflammation is involved in the pathogenesis of macular degeneration and dry eye syndrome, omega-3 is effective by suppressing the biosynthesis of arachidonic acid-derived eicosanoids (omega-6), which are proinflammatory. (13) High dietary intakes of omega-3 were associated with reduced incidence of nuclear cataract. (14) Omega-3 has a positive effect on both type 1 and 2 diabetes by reducing insulin resistance and triglycerides and increasing HDL, but it has no noticeable effect on blood glucose levels. At least two servings a week of omega-3 containing food or supplement are recommended for good health maintenance.

Spinach, kale, collards, and green beans are good sources of the carotenoids, lutein, and zeaxanthin, which have been shown to be effective in modulating macular degeneration cataract progression and color vision dynamics. Lutein and zeaxanthin are macular pigment xanthophylls that protect the retina from oxidative stress by absorbing blue light and preventing it from causing photochemical damage. Lutein inhibits nNOS and COX-2 enzyme expression in protecting the neural retina cells from ischemic death. (15) (16) (17) Daily intake should include three to five servings.

What is the role of nutrition in cataract prevention?

A diet high in processed foods, smoking, excess alcohol intake, and presence of diabetes and other chronic diseases greatly contribute to the probability of early and complicated cataract formation. Inflammatory oxygen free radicals cause the lens proteins to congeal and clump together, which leads to lens opacification.

Garlic, onions, shallots, and capers are rich in sulfur compounds, which produce an antioxidant, glutathione that may be involved in the reduction of cataract formation; and also thiacremonone, which has anti-inflammatory properties. Glutathione is made up of three amino acids: Cysteine, glycine and glutamic acid. (18) (19)

Eggs are a rich source of similar sulfur-containing compounds, as well as cysteine, lecithin, and lutein. Asparagus, broccoli, avocados, garlic, onions, spinach, and strawberries boost the liver's ability to produce glutathione. Supplements like N-acetyl cysteine, alpha lipoic acid, and vitamin C also may encourage production. Other antioxidants that can protect lens cells against free radicals include vitamins A and E, beta-carotene, lutein, lycopene, and selenium.

Soy is low in fat and high in protein. In addition to essential fatty acids, phytoestrogens, and vitamin E, it has genistein, a tyrosine-kinase inhibitor, which reduces inflammation associated with diabetes by interfering with inflammatory signaling in activated microglia. (20)

Colored fruit and vegetables like carrots, sweet potatoes, cantaloupe, papaya, grapefruit, tomatoes, pumpkins, and squash are nutritional antioxidants. They are loaded with vitamins A, C, E, and beta-carotene, which are essential for normal vision and retinal function. Vitamin A deficiency is associated with xerophthalmia and degeneration of retinal cells (rods) that lead to night blindness. Vitamin C deficiency is linked with cataract formation, normal-tension glaucoma, and macular degeneration through oxidative stress. Vitamin E appears to have some protective effect on age-related macular degeneration. (21) (22) (23) (24) (25) One clinical trial showed no appreciable effect on cataract from long-term use of vitamin C and E supplements. Most positive results come from animal trials and long-term use of whole foods in humans. (26)

Blueberries, raspberries, cranberries, strawberries, bilberries, and cherries contain anthocyanins, which are powerful anti-inflammatants in preserving retinal and macular cells. However, several studies failed to show a positive correlation with night vision and dark adaptation. (27) (28) Bilberry extract may be beneficial for the physiological renewal and homeostasis of corneal epithelial cells, but may not be as effective in macular physiology as previously posited. (29)

The polyphenol, resveratrol, in red wine and red grapes reduces oxidative stress and protects against retinal pigment epithelium hyperproliferation by inhibiting mitogen-activated kinase and extracellular signal-regulated kinase. It has been shown to have protective properties against ARMD. (30) (31)

High fructose corn syrup (sodas, ketchup, sweetened drinks)	Saturated, Trans, Hydrogenated fats (deep-fried)	Polyunsaturated vegetable oils (corn, safflower, coconut oil)	Triglycerides	Omega-6 (n-6) fatty acids (farmed fish,
Obesity, diabetes	Inflammation, myopia, AMD	Inflammation	Obesity, AMD, diabetes	Inflammation, neuropathy

Table 2: Worst Foods and their Associated Morbidities.

High-fructose corn syrup in the diet is linked to diabetes, hypertension, obesity, and their subsequent effects on vision. Its widespread use and incorporation in much of our food provides its contribution to these metabolic syndromes. Unlike glucose, fructose does not stimulate insulin secretion and its hepatic metabolism favors lipogenesis.

(32) (33) (34) (35)

A diet high in fats can lead to accumulation of plaque in blood vessel walls, including those supplying the macula, which may lead to reduction on blood flow and subsequent cell damage. Foods high in monounsaturated and polyunsaturated fats and linoleic acid were associated with a greater risk of advanced ARMD. In addition, high-saturated fat and cholesterol intake were associated with longer axial length (myopia) in eyes of healthy Singaporean Chinese children. (36) (37) (38)

Fatty acids, particularly, linoleic acid (LA) can stimulate RPE cells to express proinflammatory genes (COX-2 and iNOS), which may contribute to the pathogenesis of ARMD. The role of unsaturated fatty acids in the production of abnormal meibomian gland secretions that may lead to ocular surface abnormalities, chalazia, and possible carcinogenic disease should be investigated. Intake of foods that favor production of omega-6 polyunsaturated-derived eicosanoid fatty acids found in the typical western diet are associated with inflammatory and neurodegenerative diseases linked to overproduction of arachidonic acid. (39) (40) (41) (42)

High levels of triglycerides in the diet are associated with glucose intolerance of diabetes, microaneuryms of diabetic retinopathy, hypercholesterolemic plaque formation in small and large vessels, proliferation of inflammatory cells, and age-related macular degeneration. (43) (44)

Gluten sensitivity usually associated with celiac disease and childhood allergies, has been linked to type 2 diabetes and uveitis through its stimulation of proinflammatory cells (macrophages). (45)

Zinc	Selenium	CoenzymeQ10	Turmeric	Ginger
Green tea	Quercetin	Lutein	Anthocyanins	Beta-carotene

Table 3: Best Supplemental Antioxidants in the Diet for Eye Health

Supplements are not a substitute for good whole food.

Use high-quality antioxidant supplements in addition to good quality diet.

Read the labels.

It makes sense to eat right and exercise regularly.

A diet rich in antioxidants offers protection and repair at the cellular level, prevention of plaque adherence to blood vessel walls, and proper functioning of the immune system defenses. Its relation to the prevention of age-related cataract and macular degeneration is well documented. Observational experimental studies generally support the role of antioxidants in prevention of disease and promotion of healthy cells. Preliminary results of the TOZAL study showed that a majority of patients with dry macular degeneration had positive visual acuity outcomes when treated with a nutritional antioxidant supplement. (46) (47) (48)

Zinc is an antioxidant that is effective in slowing the progression of intermediate and advanced age-related macular degeneration. It has been shown to restore night vision in zinc deficient individuals. It prevents damage from free radicals, facilitates enzymatic reactions in protein metabolism in the retina, and helps regulate gene expression. Dietary zinc can be obtained from the consumption of peas, legumes, dried beans, garbanzos, chickpeas, black-eyed peas, soy, or supplement (10–15 mg). (49) (50) (51)

Selenium is a trace mineral that activates the antioxidant enzyme, glutathione peroxidase, which along with others, is essential for processing selenoproteins. Though it has been noted that individuals with the highest blood levels of selenium (along with vitamins C and E) have a lower risk of developing macular degeneration, there is not experimental or empirical evidence that supplementation will have a direct effect. High-blood selenium appeared to be protective for macular degeneration and cataracts associated with mercury toxicity. Dietary sources of selenium are Brazil nuts, tuna, cod, beef, spaghetti, turkey, chicken, and supplement (25 mcg). (52) (53)

Coenzyme Q10 improves the use of oxygen in the mitochondria, thereby providing more energy at the cellular level. It had a protective effect on selenite induced cataracts by reducing the oxidative stress that damages cell membranes. It also protected the lens epithelium cells from UV radiation. Coenzyme Q10 deficiency was found to be associated with cardiac and neurodegenerative diseases. Dietary coenzyme Q10 can be obtained from organ meats (60–100 mg), or by supplement in the form of ubiquinol for maximum absorption (50 mg). (54) (55)

Turmeric, whose active ingredient, curcumin, has been shown to be a powerful antioxidant and natural COX-2 inhibitor protecting retinal cells from free radical damage of light and oxidant-stress, protects the liver from toxic substances, reduces platelet aggregation, improves circulation, and reduces the acute inflammation response in anterior uveitis, autoimmune and neurodegenerative diseases. Dietary turmeric as a food additive and supplement can be obtained from mustard and curry. Amounts of 400–600 mg are adequate. (56) (57)

Ginger is another anti-inflammatory antioxidant that has been associated with a delay in the development of cataract in diabetic rats through its antiglycating activity. [6]-gingerol, an active ingredient of ginger, has antitumor, anti-inflammatory, and anti-bacterial activities that may be effective against angiogenesis-dependent diseases. (58) (59)

Green tea exerts an indirect protective effect on the eyes. Its active ingredients are polyphenols, especially epigallocatechin which reduces platelet aggregation, improves cholesterol profile, lowers blood pressure, and stimulates immune system cells to reduce inflammation and prevent infection. It may have a positive therapeutic effect on the inflammatory component of dry eye. High-quality green tea can be obtained directly in the dried leaf form (50 mg daily). (60) (61)

Quercetin is a bioflavonoid antioxidant, which inhibits the release of histamine from mast cells and blocks calcium influx across cell membranes, thereby reducing the allergic reaction and the inflammation response. It inhibits sorbitol accumulation in the lens of the eye, which leads to cataract formation and protects the retinal pigment epithelial cells from the oxidative stress effects of ultraviolet radiation. Quercetin protects the RPE in mice through direct inhibition of apoptotic pathways, but only in early pathogenesis and in a dose-dependent manner. It has a potentiating role in the prevention of oxidative degradation of vitamin C. Dietary quercetin is found in apples, citrus fruit, onions, red grapes, buckwheat, dark leafy greens, and supplement (5–10 mg) (62) (63) (64)

Lutein is a carotenoid that is found along with zeaxanthin, in high concentrations in the macular pigments. Lutein exhibits an early neuroprotective effect by inhibiting the expression of proinflammatory genes induced by linoleic acid through the blockade of NF-kB activation. It also protects the retina from damage caused by excessive UV radiation and lowers the risk of macular degeneration and cataracts. Dietary lutein and zeaxanthin can be obtained from spinach, collards, kale, romaine, peas, berries, and supplement (2–10 mg). (65) (66)

Anthocyanins are the active flavonoid ingredients of most berries. On exposure to excessive UV light, these antioxidants were shown to be protective of photo-damage rabbit retinas and against uveitis in mice through its free radical neutralization activity and inhibition of destructive inflammatory pathways. These effects include anti-allergenic, anti-viral, ant-proliferative, anti-microbial, anti-carcinogenic, microcirculatory improvement and diabetes prevention activities. A study done with anthocyanins was inconclusive for the restoration of impaired night vision. Dietary intake of grapes, blueberries, bilberry, cranberries, strawberry, blackberry, raspberry, and supplement (25 mg) are good sources. (67) (68) (69) (70)

Beta-carotene and retinal in vitamin A have been shown to be essential in the normal function of the visual purple, rhodopsin, with the resulting photochemical products stimulating the visual cells to produce an image as well as ingredients for synthesis of the corneal surface. A deficiency of these substances led to night blindness and keratomalacia. Consumption of food-based antioxidants with beta-carotene (and lutein and zeaxanthin) was associated with low risk for development of macular degeneration and cataracts. Beta-carotene supplementation may increase lung cancer incidence in smokers. Dietary intake of liver, milk, eggs, dark leafy greens, fortified cereals, carrots, cantaloupes, and supplement (2000–10,000 IU) should provide a sufficient amount of beta-carotene. (71) (72) (73) (74)

Superoxide dismutase (SOD)	Grapeseed extract (resveratrol)	Pine bark extract (pycnogenol)
N-acetyl cysteine	Ginseng extract	Cactus

Table 4: Super Antioxidants in the Diet for Eye Health

Superoxide dismutase (SOD) is an enzyme which yields glutathione and catalase and revitalizes cells and reduces rate of cell destruction by protecting against free radical oxidation from a superoxide. Glutathione counteracts the crosslinking effects and cellular damage and catalase breaks down hydrogen peroxide. Both are reactive in enhancing immune function, detoxifying heavy metals, and deactivating lipid peroxidation in the prevention and treatment of degenerative diseases, including age-related cataract formation. Food sources of SOD include honeydew melon, cantaloupe, and those containing zinc, copper, and manganese (calf's liver, crimini mushrooms, spinach, chard, asparagus, berries, oats, brown rice, and green beans). A high concentration of wheat, corn, and soy sprouts destroy the SOD molecule. (75)

Grapeseed extract has the active antioxidants proanthocyanin and resveratrol, which inhibit key components of oxidative stress and cell signaling, associated with cataractogenesis. It protects the lens epithelium by inducing the release of three antioxidative enzymes: Catalase, superoxide dismutase, and heme oxygenase. It improves small-vessel blood flow and reduces clotting time in protecting against retinal neoascularization. GSE is derived from red grapes and is now included by popular demand in energy drinks, vegetarian mayonnaise, salad dressings, and nutrition bars. (76) (77) (78)

Pine bark extract contains the vasoprotective antioxidant, *pycnogenol,* which improves retinal blood flow and stimulates improvement in retinal edema. It supports the utilization of lutein and zeaxanthin and its use in early diabetic retinopathy has been shown to have a protective effect. (79) (80)

N-acetylcysteine has been reported to help prevent the degenerative changes in the lens that leads to cataract. It helped prevent retinal detachment from contraction of collagen gel and cell proliferation in advanced diabetic vitreoretinopathy, protected the retinal pigment epithelium from effects of chronic oxidative stress in ARMD, and reduced itching symptoms from meibomian gland dysfunction. The effectiveness of a supplement in drop form in human eyes is being tested. Sources of N-acetylcysteine include yogurt, ricotta cheese, wheat germ, granola, oat flakes, and other high-protein foods. (81) (82) (83) (84)

Red ginseng (Chinese panax ginseng), acting as a retinal neural antagonist, improved the visual processes by increasing the delivery of 11 CIS-retinal from RPE to the outer disc of the photoreceptors, which resulted in decreased rhodopsin regeneration time. It may have a role in treating or preventing ocular disease. (85)

Vitamin Deficiencies and the Eye

For people over the age of fifty-five, macular degeneration is the leading cause of new severe vision loss in both the United States and Europe. It is associated with the same oxidative stress and free radical damage that causes cataract formation. High-risk factors include nutritional deficiencies, reduced gastrointestinal absorption, atherosclerosis, hypertension, environmental toxins (cigarette smoke), excessive UV radiation and infrared light damage, and aging. The photoreceptors of the retina (and the crystalline lens) have high concentrations of lipids (PUFAs) in their membranes which are prone to peroxidation due to the high oxygen tension in the outer retina. As a precaution, the retina contains a high concentration of vitamin E and C, and macular carotenoids which retard and neutralize light-induced oxidative damage. Together with retinal from vitamin A, they act in an integrated manner to protect the retina. Infants with less mature retinas and reduced efficiency of immune protective systems, may be more susceptible to oxidation than the elderly.

Case Scenario Two: A 57–year-old gentleman presents with gradual and progressive loss of central vision and cataracts that appear more advanced than normally seen at that age. Though hypertensive, he does not use the prescribed medications and does not routinely check his blood pressure. He is manifestly undernourished, smokes a pack and a half of cigarettes per day and drinks three to four scotch and sodas after work each day and admits to more on the weekends. Living alone, he eats canned food and frozen dinners but only when hungry. Suffering from frequent heartburn and nightly indigestion, he takes over-the-counter liquids, which offer some relief. After cataract surgery to both eyes, his vision improved but not as significantly as the patient had hoped. Both maculae showed degenerative changes not consistent with his age. There was no family history of similar blindness. Blood levels of B vitamins, ascorbic acid, and folates were below normal.

Vitamin C	Vitamin E	Vitamin D	Vitamin B1
Vitamin B2 (riboflavin)	Vitamin B6 (panthothenic acid)	Vitamin B12 (cobalamin)	Vitamin B9 (folic acid) *

Table 5: Vitamins for Healthy Eyes

*Though not an antioxidant itself, vitamin A discussed previously with antioxidants in its active forms as beta-carotene and retinal.

Vitamin C (ascorbic acid) is a primary antioxidant active in the repair and regeneration of tissues. It is anti-inflammatory in lowering C-reactive protein and boosts the immune system against oxidative stress. It is associated with increased efficiency in wound healing. However, supplementation with vitamin C has shown less effect on cataract progression or age-related macular degeneration. In a recent study, normal-tension glaucoma patients were found to have lower serum levels of vitamin C (and increased levels of uric acid) than control groups. Dietary sources include citrus fruit, melons, tomatoes, potatoes, broccoli, acerola, guava, and supplements (500–1000 mg). (86) (87) (88) (89)

Vitamin E is a powerful antioxidant that protects the cell membranes of blood vessels and has shown a beneficial effect on lipid peroxidation in retinal ganglion cells in experimental glaucoma in rats. However, when used alone such as in a randomized trial on humans, it has shown neither beneficial nor harmful effects on the risk of ARMD. Vitamin E in the form of alpha-tocopherol appeared to better exert its antioxidant protective and preventive effects on age-related eye disease when taken in conjunction with other antioxidants. Dietary sources of vitamin E are soy, green leafy vegetables, fish, wheat germ, nuts, seeds, and supplement (400–800 IU). (90) (91) (92)

Vitamin B1 (thiamine) deficiency in lake trout fry resulted in severe reduction in visual acuity, possibly due to reduction in carbohydrate metabolism and nerve transmission and may be correlated with nutritional deficiency seen in excessive alcohol abuse in humans. Dietary thiamine is found in fortified breads, cereals, whole grains, pasta, nuts, red meat, and supplements (1.5 mg). (93)

Vitamin B2 (riboflavin) is a cofactor for the antioxidant enzyme, glutathione reductase, and its deficiency has been associated with cataracts in both animals and humans. Supplementation studies have shown mixed results in reporting protection against cataracts in older individuals. B2 was effective in corneal cross-linkage procedures to halt the progression of keratoconus. (1.7 mg) (94) (95) (96)

Vitamin B6 (pyridoxine) deficiency (along with folate and B12) appeared to be associated with elevated levels of serum homocysteine in cases of pseudoexfoliation glaucoma and Alzheimer's disease. It inhibited glycation reactions by blocking oxidative degradation and scavenging for toxic carbonyl products of glucose and lipid degradation, making it potentially useful in the prevention and treatment of diabetic neuropathy. Dietary sources of pyridoxine include fortified cereals, fruit, beans, tuna, meat, poultry, fish, and supplements (2 mg). (97) (98)

Vitamin B12 (cobalamin) and B9 (folic acid) deficiencies have been associated with high levels of homocysteine, central retinal vein occlusion, and nutritional optic neuropathy with and without tobacco smoking and alcohol abuse. Isolated cases of eye movement disorders and loss of vision which improved with administration of cobalamin have been reported. Dietary sources of vitamin B12 and folates include oranges, lentils, cereals, leafy greens, bananas, tuna, and supplements (500 mcg/d and 100 mcg). (99) (100) (101) (102)

Vitamin D is essential in the process of immune modulation in protecting the skin and surface of the eye, prevention of microbial, viral and fungal infections, and progression of wound healing. Adequate levels are required for vitamin A absorption and assimilation. Deficient levels (<25nmol/l) were found in a higher percentage of individuals at the end of winter, more frequently among obese participants and in those with black hair, dark/olive skin, and brown eyes. Levels were higher in all individuals with more sun exposure time. Type 1 diabetes, systemic lupus erthematosus, Behçet's disease, polymyositis, rheumatoid arthritis, tuberculosis, and certain pneumonias have all been associated with deficiencies in vitamin D and supplementation may be indicated. Calcitrol (Vitamin D3) is an inhibitor of retinal neovacularization and may be of benefit in the treatment of a number of eye diseases.

Dietary sources of vitamin D include sunshine, oily fish, egg yolks, yogurt, cereals, fortified drinks, and supplements (400–1000 IU). (103) (104) (105) (106)

Good nutrition is essential to the healthy maintenance of all organ systems.

In a recent Indian study, a dietary deficiency of antioxidants and vitamins (beta-carotene, vitamin C, folic acid, iron, phytate and polyphenols) led to an increase in oxidative stress reactions in the blood and tears of cataract patients. (107)

Johanna Seddon, MD and her group at Massachusetts Eye and Ear Infirmary concluded that adequate consumption of dietary carotenoids, vitamins C, A and E when taken together as whole foods, may decrease the risk of developing advanced or exudative age-related macular degeneration. (108)

It should be noted that individuals for whom junk food, which is devoid of healthy_nutrients, is a major part of the diet are more prone to insulin-resistant diabetes and iron-deficiency retinal ischemia. Adults with tobacco/alcohol amblyopia will also have notable vitamin deficiencies. On the other hand, supplemental vitamins and herbs are used by a significant number of patients (46 percent) in a comprehensive USA setting. Ophthalmologists should systematically inquire about their use and be prepared to discuss and instruct their patients regarding concerns about the benefits and risks. (109)

Extremes:

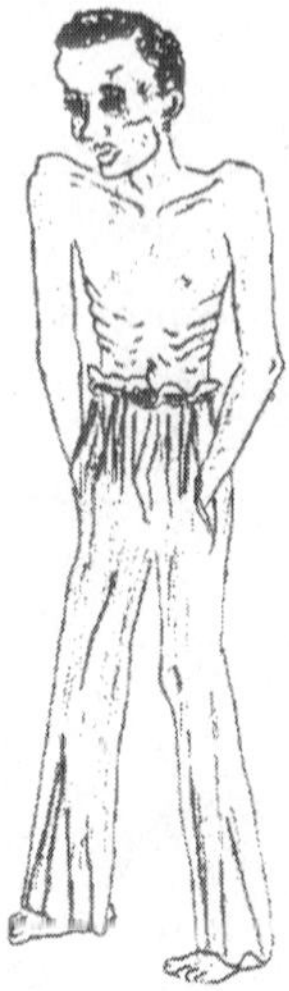

malnutrition & vitamin deficiency

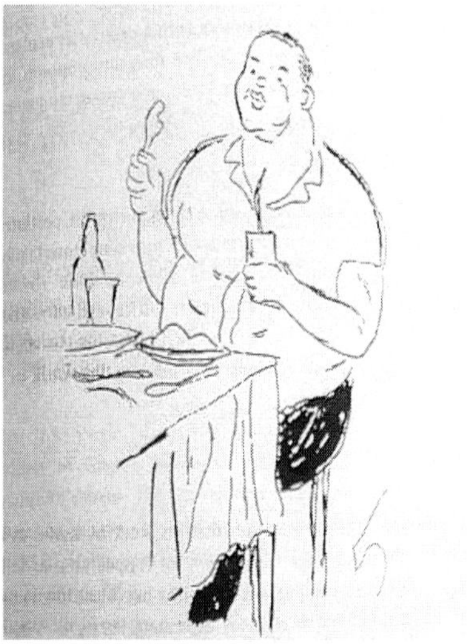

obesity from over-eating

Case Scenario Three: GS is a 48-year-old single school teacher who presented with a history of headaches, occasional tinnitus, and blurred vision, which were relieved with oral acetazolamide. Papilledema was present in both eyes, intracranial pressures were borderline normal, and her MRI was normal. She was obese and had not lost any weight in the past year over, which the papilledema had lessened and the vision had cleared substantially. She was content to keep routine follow-up appointments and use the tablets whenever she experienced tension or symptoms.

*Adapted from Medical Terminology of the Eastern Caribbean

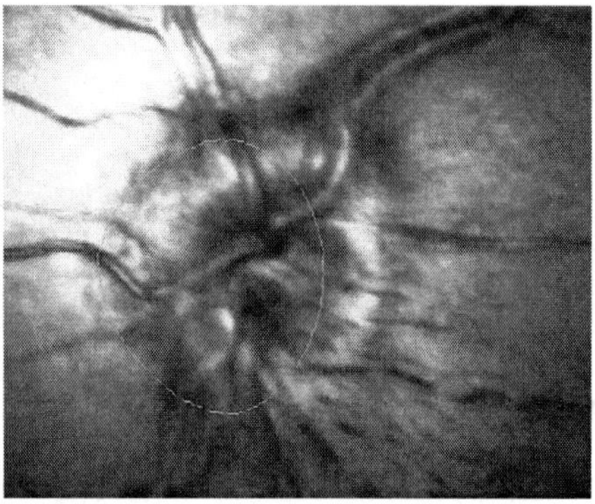

pseudotumor cerebri with papilledema

There is an established association between obesity and idiopathic intracranial hypertension (IIH) with papilledema and visual symptoms. When excessive caloric intake, lack of physical activity and emotional stress combine to create obesity, many other factors become involved. The interaction of diet, energy balance, and psychological stress with concomitant increase in glucocorticoid release can greatly affect metabolic and neuro-ophthalmic regulatory factors. Medical treatment consists of sodium-restricted weight reduction and acetazolamide. Surgery may involve optic nerve sheath fenestration and CSF shunting.

Currently, upwards of 30 percent of American adults are obese. Obesity is a well-known risk factor for type 2 diabetes, hypertension, osteoarthritis, and several cancers. It has been found to be associated with changes in lipoprotein profile, increased oxidative stress, and inflammation, which may lower the concentration of lutein and zeaxanthin in the retinal circulatory system and lead to ARMD. (110) (111) 112) (113) (114)

Weight control through good nutrition and regular exercise makes good sense.

Wine and Caffeine and the Eye

Moderate wine consumption in healthy individuals without preexisting cardiovascular pathology, either alone or in combination with beer or liquor, had a negative association with ARMD. The phenolic antioxidant, resveratrol, acts as a modulator of ischemia/reperfusion in the presence of myocardial damage, inhibitor of LDL oxidation, and suppressor of platelet aggregation. It should be noted that heavy consumption of alcohol (three or more drinks a day) is associated with increased risk of early AMD, though this may be compounded with smoking. (115) (116) (117)

Micromolar amounts of topical caffeine, through its ability to prevent oxidative stress and maintain tissue metabolic and transport functions, has been found to be effective in inhibiting the formation of galactose cataract. In its capacity to reduce glucose uptake, caffeine has been shown to have a protective effect on type 2 diabetes. The active ingredient, chlorogenic acid, can inhibit inflammation, thereby having an indirect effect on the risk of blindness. (118) (119)

Case Scenario Four: "I am 50 years old and I am interested in staying healthy and keeping good vision into my old age. You've told me what foods, supplements, and vitamins are good for my eyes, but how and when should I take them and what side effects are there?"

The best way to eat fruit is on an empty stomach. Fruit becomes alkaline and *rots* in the stomach when mixed with other food. Best times are as a midmorning snack, in-between meals, or before a meal. When fruit is cooked, the vitamin content is destroyed.

Vitamins (polyphenols, beta-carotene, anthocyanins) are best utilized when eaten *raw*, as with carrots, peas, spinach, broccoli, and red and blue fruits and vegetables. With fat-soluble vitamins and many antioxidants, excessive heat breaks down the cell walls, thereby releasing their active contents into the juices in the pan, which may be altered or discarded. The carotenoid levels in carrots, zucchini, and broccoli are released when they are boiled. When olive oil is added to avocado; lutein, lycopenes, and beta-carotenes are released.

The best time to take most supplements is after a meal, since they are absorbed better when combined with other foods. Vitamins and minerals are most effective when taken at regular intervals during the day. As many minerals are necessary for the proper absorption of vitamins, it is best to take them together. Water-soluble vitamins (B complex and C) are best taken after meals, and fat-soluble vitamins (A, C, and E) are best taken with food. Vitamin C gives an energy boost, so it may be more effective to take it in the morning. With fish oil and omega-3 supplements, the time of day does not matter, though they are best taken with food. Coenzyme Q10 is difficult to absorb and is best taken with some kind of fat or oil.

Supplements (and botanicals) should be taken consistently, as it usually takes two to three months to feel positive effects. Dosages should be regular, but it is okay to take them for two to three months, followed by two to three weeks off or similar combination.

A regimen should be chosen that is tailored to individual needs. Only high-quality phytonutrients and antioxidants should be taken. Most importantly, your physician must be kept informed of whatever supplements are being taken.

Recommendations for Healthy Eye Care:

Complimentary Nutritional Recommendations to patients >50 year old with healthy eyes:

Foods with:

Omega-3 fish oils	1000 mg twice a week
Vitamin C	500 mg daily
Lutein	2 mg
Zeaxanthin	1 mg
Zinc	20 mg
B vitamins	Complex
Bilberry (or equivalent)	30 mg
Antioxidant-rich diet with fruits & leafy greens	3–5 servings daily

Multivitamin when travelling or unable to eat a balanced diet

Annual eye exam

Complimentary Nutritional Recommendations to patients >50 year old with eye condition(s) and/or risk factors:

Foods with:

Omega-3 fish oils plus Supplements (DHA and EPA)	1000 mg daily

Multivitamin with:

Vitamin C	1000mg
Lutein	6–10mg
Zeaxanthin	3 mg
Zinc	30 mg
B vitamins	Complex
Bilberry (or equivalent)	100 mg

And

Antioxidant foods with fresh fruits and dark leafy greens	5–7 servings daily
Biannual or quarterly eye exams as per ophthalmologist	
Discuss dietary requirements and supplementation with physician(s)	
Medical and surgical eye care as indicated	

Though skeptics take great strides to refute the role of any management regimens to prevent or support eye health, other than surgery or pharmaceuticals, there is no doubt that good nutrition plays a prominent role in maintaining healthy vision. The ocular system consists of all tissue types that require basic nutrients for optimal function. The reasonable use of antioxidants and supplementation has been shown to benefit those individuals who do not meet their nutritional requirements or who are prone to certain diseases of aging, exposure and toxicity. The consumption of good, whole antioxidant-rich foods with lutein, zeaxanthin, omega-3 oils, vitamins C, A, E, and zinc remains the best practical way to avoid or minimize the risk of ARMD.

Complications of Vitamins and Supplements:

One of the obvious dangers of taking supplements lies in the possibility of mislabeled ingredients and the provision of low-quality products. There is also the possibility of overdosing, as absolute levels of safety have not been set nor are they consistent on an individual basis. Prescription drugs and supplements may be incompatible or additive in effect, as in the case of anticoagulant use. When combined with supplements like glucosamine, garlic, EPA fish oil, ginger, *Ginkgo biloba*, licorice, and vitamin E, the effect is increased and frank bleeding may occur.

Excess vitamin A is associated with pseudotumor cerebri and should be avoided in pregnancy, liver disease, and in heavy alcohol drinkers. (120) (121)

Beta-carotene has been linked with increased risk of lung cancer in smokers, through possible interactions with carcinogens causing alterations in retinal cell metabolism and signaling pathways, interactions with CYP enzymes and prooxidation/ DNA oxidation. (122) (123)

Zinc in high doses is associated with genitourinary complications. (124)

Vitamin E was associated with a small increased risk of lung cancer. (125)

Along with vitamin A and beta-carotene, excess vitamin E may actually increase all mortality, according to the Cochrane Database Systemic Review. (126)

Vitamin D in high doses has been shown to be an accelerator of atherosclerotic calcification in the elderly. (127)

References for Chapter Five:

1. Pache M, Flammer J. Surv Ophthalmol. 2006 May-Jun; 51(3): 179-212A sick eye in a sick body? Systemic findings in primary open-angle glaucoma.
2. Reiter RJ, Manchester LC, Tan DX. Curr Neuropharmacol. 2010 Sep; 8(3); 194-210.Neurotoxins: free radical mechanisms and melatonin protection.
3. Fletcher AE. Ophthalmic Res. 2010;44(3):191- Free radicals, antioxidants and eye diseases: evidence from epidemiological studies on cataract and age-related macular degeneration.
4. Age-Related Eye Disease Study Research Group. Arch Ophthalmol. 2008 Sep; 126(9):1251. A randomized, placebo-controlled, clinical triel of high-dose supplementation with vitamins C and E, beta carotene, and zinc for age-related macular degeneration and vision loss: AREDS report no. 8.
5. Krishnadev N, Meleth AD, Chew EY. Curr Opin Ophthalmol. 2010 May; 21(3): 184-9. Nutritional supplements for age-related macular degeneration.

6. NIH State-of-the-Science Conference Statement on Multivitamin/MineralSupplements and Chronic Disease Prevention. [no authors listed] NIH Consens State Sci Statements. 2006 May 15-17; 23(2):1-30.
7. Dickinson A. Filoterapia. 2011 Jan; 82(1): 5-10. History and overview of DSHEA.
8. Wong IY, Koo SC, Chan CW. Int Ophthalmol. 2011 Feb;31(1):73-82. Prevention of age-related macular degeneration.
9. Kook D, et al. Invest Ophthalmol Vis Sci. 2008 Apr; 49(4):1712-20. The protective effect of quercetin against oxidative stress in the human RPE in vitro.
10. Cortina MS, Bazan HE. Curr Opin Clin Nutr Metab Care. 2011 Mar; 14(2): 132- 7 Docosahexaenoic acid, protectins and dry eye.
11. Cakiner-Egilmez T. Insight. 2008 Oct-Dec; 33(4): 20-5. Omega-3 fatty acids and the eye.
12. Tan JS, et al.Arch Ophthalmol. 2009 May; 127(5):656-65. Dietary fatty acids and the 10-year incidence of age-related macular degeneraton: Blue Mountains Eye Study.
13. Bretillon L, et al. Exp Eye Res. 2008 Dec; 87(6): 521-8. Lipid and fatty acid profile of the retina, retinal pigment epithelium/choroid, and the lacrimal gland, and associations with adipose tissue fatty acids in human subjects.
14. McDaniel JC, Massey K, Nicolaou A. Wound Repair Regen. 2011 Mar; 19(2): 189-200. Fish oil supplementation alters levels of lipid mediators of inflammation in microenvironment of acute human wounds.
15. Townsend BS, et al. Am J Ophthalmol. 2007 Jun; 143(6): 932-939. Dietary macronutrient intake and five-year incident cataract: the blue mountains eye study.
16. Barker FM 2nd, et al. Invest Ophthalmol Vis Sci. 2011 Jan 18. Nutritional Manipulation of Primate Retinas. V: Effects of Lutein, Zeaxanthin and n-3 Fatty Acids on Retinal Sensitivity to Blue Light Damage.
17. Choi JS, et al. Nutrition. 2006 Jun; 22(6): 668-71. Inhibition of nNOS and COX-2 expression by lutein in acute retinal ischemia.

18. Ban JO, et al. Arthritis Res Ther. 2009; 11(5): R145. Anti-inflammatory and arthritic effects of theacremononone, a novel sulfur compound isolated from garlic via inhibition of NF-kappaB.
19. Reddy VN, et al. Invest Ophthalmol Vis Sci. 2001 Dec; 42(13): 3247-55.Glutathione peroxidase-1 deficiency leads to increased nuclear light scattering,membrane damage, cataract formation in gene-knockout mice.
20. Ibrahim AS, et al. Mol Vis. 2010 Oct 8; 16:2033-42. Genistein attenuates retinal inflammation associated with diabetes by targeting ofmicroglial activation.
21. Chui CJ, Taylor A. Exp Eye Res. 2007 Feb; 84(2): 229-45 Nutritional antioxidants and age-related cataract and maculopathy.
22. Tielsch JM, Sommer A. Annu Rev Nutr. 1984; 4: 183-205 The epidemiology of vitamin A deficiency and xerophthalmia.
23. Yuki K, et al. Graefes Arch Clin Exp Ophthalmol. 2010 Feb; 248(2):243-8. Reduced-serum vitamin C and increased uric acid levels in normal tensionglaucoma.
24. Tarwadi KV, Chiplonkar SA, Agte V. Clin Nutr. 2008 Jun; 27(3): 464-72. Dietary and nutritional biomarkers of lens degeneration, oxidative stress and micronutrient inadequacies in Indian cataract patients.
25. Sadaba LM, et al. Exp Eye Res. 2008 Mar; 86(3):470-9. Antioxidant effects 0f vitamins C and E, multivitamin-mineral complex andflavonoids in a model of retinal oxidative stress: the Apo-E-deficient mouse.
26. Christen WG, et al. Arch Ophthalmol. 2010 Nov; 128(11): 1397-405.Age-related cataract in a randomized trial of vitamins E and C in men.
27. Yao N, et al. J Agric Food Chem. 2010 Apr 28; 58(8): 4731-6. Protective effects of bilberry (Vaccinium myrtillus L.) extract against endotoxin- induced uveitis in mice.
28. Levy Y, Glovinsky Y. Eye (Lond). 1998; 12 (pt 6): 967-9. The effect of anthocyanosides on night vision.
29. Song J, et al. Phytother Res. 2010 Apr; 24(4): 520-4. Protective effect of bilberry (Vaccinium myrtillus L.) extracts on cultured human corneal limbal epithelial cells (HCLEC).

30. King RE, Kent KD, Bomser JA. Chem Biol Interact. 2005 Jan 15; 151(2): 143-9. Resveratrol reduces oxidation and proliferation of human retinal pigment epithelial cells via extracellular signal-regulated kinase inhibition.
31. Sheu SJ, Liu NC, Chen JL. J Ocul Pharmacol Ther. 2010 Jun; 26(3):231-6.Resveratrol protects human retinal pigment epithelial cells from acrolein-induced damage.
32. Ferder L, Ferder MD, Inserra F. Curr Hypertens Rep. 2010 Apr; 12(2): 105-12. The role of high-fructose corn syrup in metabolic syndrome and hypertension.
33. Moeller SM, et al. J Am Coll Nutr. 2009 Dec; 28(6): 619-26The effects of high fructose syrup.
34. Tappy L, et al. Nutrition. 2010 Nov-Dec; 26(11-12): 1044-9. Fructose and metabolic diseases: new findings, new questions.
35. Bray GA, Nielsen SJ, Popkin BM. Am J Clin Nutr. 2004 Apr; 79(4):537-43.Consumption of high-fructose corn syrup in beverages may play a role in theepidemic of obesity.
36. Parekh N, et al. Arch Ophthalmol. 2009 Nov; 127(11): 1483-93. Association between dietary fat intake and age-related macular degeneration in the Carotenoids in Age-Related Eye Disease Study (CAREDS): an ancillary study of the Women's Health Initiative.
37. Seddon JM, et al. Arch Ophthalmol. 2001 Aug; 119(8): 1191-9. Dietary fat and risk for advanced age-related macular degeneration.
38. Lim LS, et al. Ophthalmology. 2010 May; 117(5):993-997. Dietary factors, myopia, and axial dimensions in children.
39. Fang IM, et al. Mol Nutr Food Res. 2009 Jun; 53(6): 739-50. Comparative effects of fatty acids on proinflammatory gene cyclogenase 2 and inducible nitric oxide synthase expression in retinal pigment epithelial cells.
40. Butovich IA. Invest Ophthalmol Vis Sci. 2011 Feb 1; 52(1):639-41.On the presence of (O-acyl)-omega-hydroxy fatty acids and of their esters in humanmeibomian gland secretions.
41. Wall R, et al. Nutr Rev. 2010 May; 68(5):280-9 Fatty acids from fish: the anti-inflammatory potential of long-chain omega-3 fatty acids.

42. Young K. Int J Food Sci Nutr. 2009; 60 Suppl 5:203-11. Omega-6 (n-6) and omega-3 (n-3) fatty acids in tilapia and human health: a review.
43. De Fine Olivarius N, et al. BMC Public Health. 2011 Feb 4; 11:80. Prevalence and progression of visual impairments in patients newly diagnosed with clinical type 2 diabetes: a 6 –year follow up study.
44. Helfenstein T, et al. Int J Exp Pathol. 2011 Feb; 92(1): 40-9. Impaired glucose tolerance plus hyperlipidaemia induced by diet promotes retina microaneurysms in New Zealand rabbits.
45. Krifa F, et al. Gastroenterol Clin Biol. 2010 Apr-May; 34(4-5):319-20. Uveitis responding on gluten free diet in a girl with celiac disease and diabetes mellitus type 1.
46. Chiu CJ, Taylor A. Exp Eye Res. 2007 Feb; 84(2):229-45. Nutritional antioxidants and age-related cataract and maculopathy.
47. Fletcher AE. Ophthalmic Res. 2010; 44(3):191-8. Free radicals, antioxidants and eye diseases: evidence from epidemiological studies on cataract and age-related macular degeneration.
48. Cangemi FE. BMC Ophthalmol. 2007 Feb 26; 7:3.TOZAL study: an open case control study of an oral antioxidant and omega-3 supplement for dry AMD.
49. Saper RB, Rash R. Am Fam Physician. 2009 May 1; 79(9): 768-72. Zinc: an essential micronutrient.
50. Newsome DA. Curr Eye Res. 2008 Jul; 33(7): 591-8. A randomized, prospective, placebo-controlled clinical trial of a novel zinc-monocysteine compound in age-related macular degeneration.
51. Christian P, et al. Am J Clin Nutr. 2001 Jun;73(6):1045-51. Zinc supplementation might potentiate the effect of vitamin A in restoring night vision in pregnant Nepalese women.
52. Flohé L. Dev Ophthalmol. 2005; 38:89-102.Selenium, selenoproteins and vision.
53. Lemire M, et al. Environ Health Perspect. 2010 Aug 17. Selenium and Mercury in the Brazilian Amazon: Opposing Influences on Age-Related Cataracts.

54. Kemt M, et al. Acta Ophthalmol. 2010 May; 88 (3):e78-86. Coenzyme Q10 prevents human lens epithelial cells from light-induced apoptotic cell death by reducing oxidative stress and stabilizing BAX / Bcl-2 ratio.
55. Siemieniuk E, Skrzydlewska E. Postepy Hig Med Dosw (Online). 2005; 59:150-9. [Coenzyme Q10: its biosynthesis and biological significance in animal organisms and in humans].
56. Aggarwal BB, Harikumar KB. Int J Biochem Cell Biol. 2009 Jan; 41(1):40-59.Potential therapeutic effects of curcumin, the anti-inflammatory agent, against neurodegenerative, cardiovascular, pulmonary, metabolic, autoimmune and neoplastic diseases.
57. Mandal MN, et al. Free Radic Biol Med. 2009 Mar 1; 46(5):672-9. Curcumin protects retinal cells from light-and-oxidant stress-induced cell death.
58. Saraswat M, et al. Mol Vis. 2010 Aug 10; 16:1525-37. Antiglycating potential of Zingiber officinalis and delay of diabetic cataract in rats.
59. Kim EC, et al. Biochem Biophys Res Commun. 2006 Sep 23; 335(2): 300-8. [6]-Gingerol, a pungent ingredient of ginger, inhibits angiogenesis in vitro and in vivo
60. Graham HN.Prev Med. 1992 May; 21(3): 334-50. Green tea composition, consumption, and polyphenol chemistry.
61. Cavet ME, et al. Mol Vis. 2011 Feb 18; 17:533-42. Anti-inflammatory and anti-oxidative effects of the green tea polyphenol epigallocatechin gallate in human corneal epithelial cells.
62. Cao X, et al. Exp Eye Res. 2010 Jul; 91(1): 15- 25. The effects of quercetin in cultured human RPE cells under oxidative stress and in Ccl2/Cx3cr1 double deficient mice.
63. Kook D, et al. Invest Ophthalmol Vis Sci. 2008 Apr; 49(4): 1712-20. The protective effect of quercetin against oxidative stress in the human RPE in vitro.
64. Beker BY, et al. Int J Food Sci Nutr. 2011 Mar 10. Protection of ascorbic acid from copper (II)-catalyzed oxidative degradation in the presence of flavonoids: quercetin, catechin and morin.

65. Li SY, et al. Invest Ophthalmol Vis Sci. 2009 Feb; 50(2):836- 43. Effect of lutein on retinal neurons and oxidative stress in a model of acute retinal ischemia/reperfusion.
66. Krinsky NI, Landrum JT, Bone RA. Annu Rev Nutr. 2003; 23:171-201.Biologic mechanisms of the protective role of lutein and zeaxanthin in the eye.
67. Liu Y, et al. J Agric Food Chem. 2011 Jan 12; 59(1): 356-63. Identification of anthocyanin components of wild Chinese blueberries and amelioration of light-induced retinal damage in pigmented rabbit using whole berries.
68. Yao N, et al. J Agric Food Chem. 2010 Apr 28; 58(8):4731-6. Protective effects of bilberry (Vaccinium myrtillus L.) extract against endotoxin-induced uveitis in mice.
69. Ghosh D, Konishi T. Asia Pac J Clin Nutr. 2007; 16(2): 200-8. Anthocyanins and anthocyanin-rich extracts: role in diabetes and eye function.
70. Canter PH, Ernst E. Surv Ophthalmol. 2004 Jan-Feb; 49(1): 38-50. Anthocyanisides of Vaccinium myrtillus (bilberry) for night vision—a systematic review of placebo-controlled trials.
71. Lanska DJ. Handb Clin Neurol. 2010; 95:435-44. Chapter 29: historical aspects of the major neurological vitamin deficiency disorders: overview and fat-soluble vitamin A.
72. Agte V, Tarwadi K. Ophthalmic Res. 2010; 44(3): 166-72. The importance of nutrition in the prevention of ocular disease with special reference to cataract.
73. Goldberg J, et al. Am J Epidemiol. 1988 Oct; 128(4):700-10. Factors associated with age-related macular degeneration. An analysis of data from first National Health and Nutrition examination Survey.
74. Albanes D, et al. J Natl Cancer Inst. 1996 Nov 6; 88(21):1560-70. Alpha-Tocopherol and beta-carotene supplements and lung cancer incidence in the Alpha-tocopherol, beta-carotene cancer prevention study: effects of base-line characteristics and study compliance.

75. Babizhayev MA. Cell Biol Funct. 2011 Mar 7.Mitochondria induce oxidative oxygen species and stress, generation of reactive oxygen species and redox state unbalance of the eye lens leading to human cataract formation: disruption of redox lens organization by phospholipid hydrperoxides as a common basis for cataract disease.
76. Barden CA, et al. Am J Vet Res. 2008 Jan; 69(1): 94-100Effect of grape polyphenols on oxidative stress in canine lens epithelial cells.
77. Zheng Y, et al. Mol Vis. 2010 Aug 4; 16: 467-74. Resveratrol protects human lens epithelial cells against H2O2-induced oxidative stress by increasing catalase, SOD-1, and HO-1 expression.
78. Hua J, et al. Invest Ophthalmol Vis Sci. 2011 Jan 31. Resveratrol Inhibits Pathological Retinal Neovascularization in Vldlr-/-Mice.
79. Steigerwalt R, et al. J Ocul Pharmacol Ther. 2009 Dec; 25(6): 537-40. Pycnogenol improves microcirculation, retinal edema, and visual acuity in early diabetic retinopathy.
80. Dene BA, et al. J Ocul Pharmacol Ther. 2005 Feb; 21(1):28-35. Effects of antioxidant treatment on normal and diabetic rat retinal enzyme activities.
81. Wang P, et al. Mol Vis. 2009 Dec 31; 15: 2945-52. Hyperoxia-induced lens damage in rabbit:protective effects of N-acetylcysteine.
82. Lei H, et al. Am J Pathol. 2010 Jul; 177(1): 132-40. N-acetylcysteine suppresses retinal detachment in an experimental model of proliferative vitreoretinopathy.
83. Gerona G, et al. J Ocul Pharmacol Ther. 2010 Aug 26(4):309-14. Antioxidants N-acetyl-cysteine protects retinal pigmented epithelial cells from long- term hypoxia changes in gene expression.
84. Akyol-Salman I, et al. J Ocul Pharmacol Ther. 2010 Aug; 26(4): 329-33. Efficacy of topical N-acetylcysteine in the treatment of meibomian gland dysfunction.
85. Wahid F, et al. Planta Med. 2010 Mar; 76(5):426-32.Effects of red ginseng extract on visual sensitivity and ERG b-wave of bullfrog'seye.
86. Desneves KJ, et al. Clin Nutr. 2005 Dec; 24(6):979-87. Treatment with supplementary arginine, vitamin C and zinc in patients with pressure ulcers: a randomized controlled trial.

87. SanGiovanni JP, et al. Arch Ophthalmol. 2007 Sep; 125(9): 1225-32.The relationship of dietary carotenoid and vitamin A, E, and C intake with age- related macular degeneration in a case-control study: AREDS Report No. 22.
88. Fernandez MM, Afshari NA. Curr Opin Ophthalmol. 2008 Jan; 19(1):66-70. Nutrition and the prevention of cataracts.
89. Yuki K, et al. Graefes Arch Clin Exp Ophthalmol. 2010 Feb; 248(2):243-8. Reduced-serum vitamin C and increased uric acid levels in normal-tension Glaucoma.
90. Ko ML, et al. Curr Eye Res. 2010 Sep; 35(9):842-9. Dietary deficiency of vitamin E aggravates retinal ganglion cell death in experimental glaucoma of rats.
91. Christen WG, et al. Ophthalmology. 2010 Jun; 117(6): 1163-8. Vitamin E and age-related macular degeneration in a randomized trial of women.
92. Jin H, et al. Med Chem. 2010 Feb 11; 53(3):1117-27. Multifunctional antioxidants for the treatment of age-related diseases.
93. Carvalho PS, et al. J Aquat Anim Health. 2009 Dec; 21(4):315-25. Thiamine deficiency effects on the vision and foraging ability of lake trout fry.
94. Sperduto RD, et al. Arch Ophthalmol. 1993 Sep; 111(9):1246-53. The Linxian cataract studies.Two nutrition intervention trials.
95. Meyer CH, Sekundo W. Dev Ophthalmol. 2005; 38:103-19. Nutritional supplementation to prevent cataract formation.
96. O'Brart DP, et al. Br J Ophthalmol. 2011 Feb 24. A randomized, prospective study to investigate the efficacy of riboflavin/ultraviolet A (370 nm) corneal cross-linkage to halt the progression of keratoconus.
97. Roedl JB, et al. J Neural Transm. 2007; 114(5):571-5.Vitamin deficiency and hyperhomocysteinemia in pseudoexfoliation glaucoma.
98. Voziyan PA, et al. Cell Mol Life Sci. 2005 Aug; 62(15): 1671-81. Pyridoxamine as a multifunctional pharmaceutical: targeting pathogenic glycationand oxidative damage.

99. Taubert M, Dowd TC, Wood A. J Med Case Reports. 2008 Mar 10; 2: 77. Malnutrition and bilateral central retinal vein occlusion in a young woman: a casereport
100. De Silva P, Jayamanne G, Bolton R. J Med Case Reports. 2008 Sep 10; 2:299. Folic acid deficiency optic neuropathy: a case report.
101. Hsu CT, Miller NR, Wray ML. Ophthalmologica. 2002 Jan-Feb; 216(1):65-7. Optic neuropathy from folic acid deficiency without alcohol abuse.
102. Veldt BJ, et al. Eur L Intern Med. 2006 Jul; 17(4): 292-4. Loss of vision as a presenting sign of cobalamin deficiency: An eye-opener.
103. Schwalfenberg GK. Mol Nutr Food Res. 2011 Jan 55(1): 96-108. A review of the critical role of vitamin D in the functioning of the immune system and the clinical implications of vitamin D deficiency.
104. Kimlin M, et al. J Photochem Photobiol B. 2007 Dec 14; 89(2-3): 139-47. Does a high UV environmental ensure adequate vitamin D status?
105. Pelajo CF, Lopez-Benitez JM, Miller LC. Autoimmun Rev. 2010 May; 9(7): 507-10.Vitamin D and autoimmune rheumatologic disorders.
106. Albert DM, et al. Invest Ophthalmol Vis Sci. 2007 May; 48(5): 2327-34.Calcitrol is a potent inhibitor of retinal neovascularization.
107. Dietary and nutritional biomarkers of lens degeneration, oxidative stress and micronutrient inadequacies in Indian cataract patients. Tarwadi KV, ChiplonkarSA, Agte V. Clin Nutr. 2008 Jun; 27(3):464-72.
108. Seddon JM, et al. JAMA. 1994 Nov 9; 272(18):1413-20. Dietary carotenoids, vitamins A, C, and E, and advanced age-related macular degeneration. Eye Disease Case-Control Studies Group.
109. West Al, et al. Am J Ophthalmol. 2005 Mar; 139(3):522-9. Herb and vitamin supplementation use among a general ophthalmology practice population.
110. Daniels AB, et al. Am J Ophthalmol. 2007 Apr; 143(4):635-41. Profiles of obesity, weight gain, and quality of life in idio[athic intracranialhypertension (pseudotumor cerebri).

111. Hannerz J, Ericson K. Headache. 2009 Feb;49(2): 178-84. The relationship between idiopathic intracranial hypertension and obesity.
112. Spencer SJ, Tilbrook A. Stress. 2011 Feb 6. The glucocorticoid contribution to obesity.
113. Wall M. Curr Neurol Neurosci Rep. 2008 Mar;8(2):87-93. Idiopathic intracranial hypertension (pseudotumor cerebri).
114. Johnson EJ. Nutr Rev. 2005 Jan; 63(1):9-15.Obesity, lutein metabolism, and age-related macular degeneration: a web of connections.
115. Obisesan TO, et al. J Am Geriatr Soc. 1998 Jan; 46(1):1-7. Moderate wine consumption is associated with decreased odds of developing age-related macular degeneration in NHANES-1.
116. Wu JM, et al. Int J Mol Med. 2001 Jul; 8(1):3-17 Mechanism of cardioprotection by resveratrol, a phenolic antioxidant present in red wine (Review).
117. Chong EW, et al. Am J Ophthalmol. 2008 Apr; 145(4):707-715. Alcohol consumption and the risk of age-related macular degeneration: a systematic review and meta-analysis.
118. Varma SD, Kovtun S, Hegde K. Mol Vis. 2010 Dec 8; 16:2626-33.Effectiveness of topical caffeine in prevention: studies with galactose cataract.
119. Kempf K, Martin S. Med Klin (Munich). 2010 Dec; 105(12):910-5. [Coffee and Diabetes].
120. Fraunfelder FW. Drugs Today (Barc). 2005 Aug; 41(8):537-45. Ocular side effects associated with dietary supplements and herbal medicines.
121. Bartlett H, Eperjesi F. Ophthalmic Physiol Opt. 2005 May; 25(3):179-94. Possible contraindications and adverse reactions associated with the use ofocular nutritional supplements.
122. Goralczyk R. Nutr Cancer. 2009 61(6):767-74. Beta-carotene and lung cancer in smokers: review of hypotheses and status of research.

123. Russell RM. J Nutr. 2004 Jan; 134(1): 262S-268S.The enigma of beta-carotene in carcinogenesis: what can be learned from animal studies.
124. Johnson AR, et al. J Urol 2007 Feb; 177(2):639-43. High dose zinc increases hospital admissions due to genitourinary complications.
125. Slatore CG, et al. Am J Respir Crit Care Med 2008 Mar; 177(5):524-30.Long-term use of supplemental multivitamins, vitamin C, vitamin E, and folate does not reduce the risk of lung cancer.
126. Bjelakovic G, et al. Cochrane Database Syst Rev. 2008 Apr 16;(2):CD007176. Antioxidant supplements for prevention of mortality in healthy participantsand patients with various diseases.
127. Hellemons ME, Bakker SJ. Diabetologia. 2010 Dec;53(12):2688. Vitamin D as an accelerator of atherosclerotic calcification: a D-tail that may be a Trojan horse.

Botanicals for the Eyes

Introduction: Herbal remedies have been used for thousands of years and in every culture known for conditions such as red eyes, vision enhancement, night blindness, allergic reactions, bacterial and viral conjunctivitis, cataracts, glaucoma, and aging vision. Modern synthetic eyedrops have been in existence for a few decades at most. The active ingredients of medicinal plants are specifically indicated for the correction of inflammation, infections, edema, tissue healing, fluid regulation and hormonal regulation, and vision deterioration due to improper blood flow. Plants contain complex interconnected phytochemicals, the foundation upon which most of our pharmaceutical drugs are based. The action of plant-based chemicals in modulating the immune system is the most important mechanism involved in disease prevention and healing.Western medicine relies heavily on evidence-based drugs, and until recently, it has rejected its own natural-based (Native American) medicine. Eastern medicine has been able to incorporate both modern research methods and traditional medicine. European medicine approaches a blend of traditional herbal and conventional medicine, a partnership which continues to be quite effective. Currently, we tend to use five main groups of drugs all of which can be plant based: Antimicrobials, anti-inflammatories, antiglaucomas, lubricants, and antivasculars. Integration of herbal medicine into clinical courses and curriculae in the west is becoming more frequent.

Though herbals are perceived as *natural and safe*, there may be misconceptions about their side effects and interactions with other *drugs*. The less regulated a substance is, the less harmful it is believed to be. However, if they are equally effective as patented drugs, the same potential for untoward effects may be present. The physician should be aware of the properties, activities, methods of blending, concepts of prevention, indications, and contraindications of the more common botanicals in widespread use today. Though relatively safe and easily available, herbal treatments should be used along with medical consultation. For eye conditions, such as blepharitis and conjunctivitis, many people prefer herbal treatments either because professional care may be inconvenient or pharmaceuticals are not readily available, or both may be too costly. Caution: Many home remedies are made without aseptic techniques. Packaging may be without adequate expiration specifications, or the product may be stored in reusable bottles without preservatives. Avoid boric acid powder mixed at home due to asepsis and possible boron toxicity. If no improvement occurs within three days, appropriate medical care is recommended.

Indications for Herbal Treatments of Red Eyes:

Minor eye irritations without discharge, congested eyes from fatigue, swimming, smog, sun glare, exposure to smoke, dry eyes without accessory symptoms, loose foreign material evident, and common allergic redness from pollen, grass, animal hair, and dust may all respond favorably to the use of demulcents, cellulose derivatives, polyvinyl alcohols, emollients, collyrium eye washes, and other sterile ocular solutions derived from botanicals.

Contraindications to Herbal Treatments for Red Eyes:

Foreign body in the cornea, corneal edema, irritation and redness from contact lens wear, any discharge in the lids or eye, follicular conjunctivitis (traditional pinkeye), pain, history of glaucoma should be evaluated and treated by professional medical care. *How and why do they work?*

Botanicals contain complex mixtures of ingredients which act at the molecular and cellular levels to enhance or inhibit chemical reactions.

Carbohydrates	Lipids	Amino acids	Phenols	Terpenes
Flavonoids	Tannins	Proanthocyanins	Coumarins	Saponins
Glycosides	Polysaccharides	Glucosilinates	Alkaloids	Lignans
Sulfurs	Resins	Sterols	Water	Vitamins/Minerals

Table 1. Active Ingredients of Medicinal Plants.* (1)

*This is a very small representative number of active ingredients of plants.

Knowledge of the chemical properties of plants is crucial to the overall understanding of how and why such chemicals interact with the human body. Phenols exhibit their anti-inflammatory action by inhibiting COX-2 enzymes in the inflammation pathway. Volatile oils are complex mixtures of terpenes with strong antiseptic, anti-inflammatory and antiallergic properties. Flavonoids are polyphenolic compounds with pigments that are essential for retinal function, maintain healthy circulation and strengthen capillary walls to prevent leakage into the surrounding tissues. Tannins are astringents, with binding properties which help in preventing bleeding and leakage, and proanthocyanins provide antioxidant protection against free radical damage.

Coumarins are anti-inflammatory, antiseptic blood thinners. Saponins provide steroidal activity in modulating immune reactions. Some glycosides provide diuretic action in regulating fluid balance and others have sedative and relaxant effects. Polysaccharides have immune system activity and glucosilinates are useful in increasing blood flow to tissues when needed. Alkaloids are important in providing cycloplegia (atropine), relieving pain, reducing spasms and drying up body secretions. Their effects on the central nervous system can be regulatory or intoxicating. Lignans are polyphenolic phytoestrogens which act as antioxidants capable of interfering with the cancer-promoting effects of estrogen in breast cancer. Resins include gums, terpenoids, and phenols which have a protective effect on the plant and may be toxic to predators. Sterols are a mixture of steroid alcohols and vitamin D precursors, which have a regulatory effect on cholesterol and other vegetable oils in arterial blood vessels. The antibacterial agent, allicin, from garlic and onions, contains 40 percent oxygenated allyl sulfur. Plants contain numerous vitamins and minerals essential to the function of healthy tissue. The water content of living cells is essential to creation and maintenance of all the properties of plants through active transport, diffusion, osmosis, and plasmolysis.

Advantages of Botanicals Over Drugs:

Scientific methods cannot provide all the answers, particularly in and of the human body. Synthesized drugs cannot balance and regulate a system like a complex group of phytochemicals. Botanicals may be slower in action for acute conditions such as alleviation of pain and inflammation, but have a clear advantage in having a lower potential for side effects and a broader range of possible actions. In many cases, the mechanism of action of the plant is to correct the underlying cause of the illness and not just reduce its symptoms.

Death and serious injury from FDA-approved drugs in 2009 came to 63,846 and 373,535. Drug side effects are the nation's fourth leading cause of death. (2) However, there were zero deaths attributed to herbs, supplements, vitamins, and amino acids. (3)

Under current FDA laws, herbs are considered supplements, not drugs. They are not intended to diagnose, treat, cure, or prevent any disease processes. They are, however, intended to assist healing. They do not and will not be able to compete with standard medical therapies unless there is a drastic change in pharmaceutical regulation, standardization, and funding for these products, as well as changes in the public's overall perception of medicine. Botanicals can treat chronic diseases such as arthritis and asthma that cannot be treated by pharmaceuticals without the increased risk of serious side effects.

Botanicals are more economical than synthetic drugs, and in some cases, they may be more environmentally friendly. Though different herbalist and naturopaths may have different regimens for the same disease, if it is applied properly to the *individual situation*, this is an advantage in that less may be better and not more which may result in detrimental side effects.

Disadvantages of Botanicals compared to drugs:

Critics maintain the belief that *botanicals are ineffective*. They take longer to work, then are as or more effective. They don't work as fast and are not as strong as drugs. Dose for dose this may be true, but rather than herbs being too weak, drugs may be too strong. *Herbs are unregulated*. There are more journal articles and closer scrutiny on herbs than on drugs. Celebrex and Vioxx escaped scrutiny and did a lot of damage before their potency was recognized by the public. Regulations on drugs have not stopped them from being dangerous. Regulation does not guarantee safety.

Herbs are unstandardized. Recent scientific methods of extraction and analysis of herbs has led to more determination of more exact quality and quantity of active ingredients in plants. Unfortunately in North America, where herbal patenting is not profitable in a health system dominated by pharmaceutical companies, a perfectly safe and efficacious plant may be overlooked despite its beneficial properties. (e.g., *Aloe vera* for wound healing).

The positives and negatives in the comparison of drugs and botanicals are currently more political than physiological. The use of botanicals by consumers is on the rise in North America as they become more aware of the potentially serious side effects of pharmaceutical drugs and the comparative benefits and safety of natural products. Though herbals are not substitutes for conventional pharmaceuticals with specific indications, physicians should be aware and have some knowledge of their existence, features and widespread use.

Case Scenario One: A 65-year-old female patient with diabetes, HBP, arthritis, and recurrent conjunctivitis; all for which prescription eyedrops irritate or burn, and therefore, doesn't take the medications. But she has eyebright growing in her garden. She asks, "What herbals are good for the eyes? And how do I take them?"

The most important thing the patient did was ask for the doctor's advice on the use of herbals for her conditions. Botanicals for eyes or other organ treatments should be taken with medical supervision and awareness.

Bilberry	Ginkgo biloba	Grapeseed	Pine bark	Saffron
Broccoli	Cabbage	Corn	Pepper	Spinach

Table 2. Botanicals for improved eyesight:
(Best ingested as whole food or herbal teas; all are evidence based)

Bilberry (*Vaccinium myrtillus*) contains anthocyanosides that trigger genetic signaling for promoting eye health and preventing disease. (4) It has shown definitive anti-inflammatory properties by preventing endotoxin-induced uveitis in mice through an increase in the expression of copper/zinc and manganese superoxide dismutase and GPX mRNA. (5) Both a protective effect through the physiological renewal and homeostasis of corneal epithelial cells (6) and a neuroprotective effect on the retina via an antioxidation mechanism (7) have been shown in both in vitro and in vivo studies. It has demonstrated a decreased rate of age-related macular degeneration (ARMD) by improving blood flow thru the capillaries, as well as increasing capillary permeability. Its anthocyanosies protect the retina from damage by upregulating oxidative stress defense enzymes, HO-1 and GST-pi in the RPE. (8) The improvement in night vision through oral administration of bilberry extract remains controversial, with most studies refuting the claim. (9) (10) It has been used to treat early diabetic retinopathy and a.m. in rat models with promising results. (11) Pretreatment with bilberry extract before the induction of hypertension has been shown to maintain the blood-brain barrier and vascular permeability through protection of the collagens in the vessel walls. Perhaps there may be a role in the improvement of hypertensive retinopathy. (12) It has been shown to reduce and prevent diabetic cataracts caused by elevation of polyols within the lens of the eye catalysed by enzyme aldose reductase. Bilberry contains flavonoids, especially quercetin and its derivatives, which are potent inhibitors of aldose reductase, a crucial enzyme in cataract formation. It is especially effective in slowing the progression of cataracts when used in conjunction with vitamin E. (13) (14)

Preparation: Eat 1 cup fresh berries daily (blueberries may be substituted) = 470 mg fruit.May be consumed in a dosage range of 360–600 mg per day as a standardized extract containing 25 percent anthocyanosides. (15) *

Caution: Bilberry in contraindicated in advanced insulin-dependent diabetes as it potentiates insulin levels and may lead to increased bleeding from coumarin-like activity.

**preparations coordinated with National Geographic Guide to Medicinal Herbs*

Ginkgo biloba (*G. biloba*) contains antioxidants for free radical protection, consisting mostly of glycosides for nerve cell protection and terpene lactones, which reduce inflammation. Its main feature of benefit in the eye is in improving circulation in small blood vessels. However, most studies show only a moderate improvement over placebo. It should be noted that placebo does exceptionally well in vascular conditions. Ginkgo has been shown to improve cognitive vascular effects in older human individuals (16) and prolong retinal ganglion cell survival in rats. (17) It promotes blood circulation to the optic nerve head, improves oxygenation and increases ocular blood flow velocity. (18) (19) It prevents steroid-induced ocular hypertension at the trabecular meshwork, (20) and has been shown to be effective against diabetic cataract. (21) Ginkgo appears to improve the visual fields in some patients with normal tension glaucoma (NTG). (22)

Future research is warranted in identifying and designating the precise role of *Ginkgo biloba* in glaucoma. (23)

Preparation: Steep one tsp dried ginkgo leaf in one cup hot water for five to seven minutes, strain, drink one to two cups daily. May be taken as a standardized extract 120 mg of 24–27 percent flavone glycosides and 6–7 percent triterpenes, bid

Caution: Due to its coumarinic activity, *Ginkgo biloba* should be used with caution in patients taking blood thinners.

Grapeseed extract (*Vitus vinifera*) is a potent antioxidant containing proanthocyanidins, which protect the lens epithelial cells from oxidative stress. In animal studies, it has been shown to suppress cataractogenesis through its attenuation of stress-induced cell signaling in HLE-B3 cells. (24) (25) (26) It has exhibited strong chemoprotective properties at the molecular level including free radical scavenging ability, antiendonucleoltic activity, cytochrome P450 2E 1 inhibitory activity, antinecrotic, antiapoptotic, and anticarcinogenic activities, as well as modulatory effects on regulatory genes. It also improves peripheral circulation in eyes, strengthens capillaries, and appears to reduce eyestrain from computer use. (27) Cumulative evidence suggests that moderate wine consumption exerts a cardioprotective effect. Through vasodilator activity from compounds in the skin of vinifera grapes, an antihypertensive action is induced, which is protective to the retinal vasculature and cells. It is rich in vitamin E, flavonoids, polyphenols, linoleic acid, and resveratrol. (28)

Preparation: May take 300–600 mg in standardized capsule or tablet form once daily for eye health. Available as tincture with drops added to water or as one serving of wine for women and 1–2 servings for men or 4–6 ounces of dark grape juice per day. May use grapeseed oil to add to salads or for cooking.

Caution: Due to the high incidence in the use of pesticides in the agriculture of grapes, toxic effects may occur. Women should be aware of the incidence of breast cancer in the excessive consumption of wine. Alcohol in contraindicated during pregnancy. Side effects include headaches, nausea, dizziness, and dry itchy scalp. It may increase the clotting time of blood.

Pine bark extract (*Pinus maritima*) is made from the bark of the French maritime pine tree, which contains proanthocyanins and oligomeric proanthrocyanidin complexes, the most prominent of which is pycnogenol, which in turn is composed mainly of procyanidins and phenolic acids. Clinical studies have confirmed that PYC is effective in the treatment of chronic venous insufficiency and retinal microhemorrhages. It protects against oxidative stress by doubling the intracellular synthesis of antioxidant enzymes and scavenging free radicals. It has a role in the protection and regeneration of vitamins C and E, and its anti-inflammatory activity has been demonstrated both in vitro and in vivo studies. (29) Its antioxidant properties have been shown to be of benefit in early diabetic retinopathy by enhancing retinal circulation by regression of edema. (30) By reducing blood vessel damage, it improved capillary resistance, reduced the accumulation of fatty deposits in retinal arteries and reduced leakage into the retina. (31) (32)

Preparation: Available in standardized capsules or tablets at 200 mg/day, recommended starting dosage, then maintained at 50–100 mg daily.

Caution: Pine bark extract has been reported to inhibit the release of histamine from mast cells. (33) It may be contraindicated in people with autoimmune conditions, due to its potential interference with drugs used to suppress the immune system. High doses may interfere with radiation or chemotherapy. It inhibits angiotensin converting enzyme (ACE) activity and can potentially interact with blood pressure-lowering medications in hypertension. (34) Mild headaches, nausea, and upset stomach have been reported.

Saffron (*Crocus sativa*) may protect the photoreceptors from retinal stress by acting as a regulator of apoptosis. The active ingredient, crocetin, is a carotenoid with an inhibitory effect against cell death induced by damaging light-released toxins in a mouse ganglion cell line. (35) It prevents retinal degeneration induced by oxidative stress by inhibition of the destructive effects of the enzyme caspase-3 and -9. (36) There is the indication that short-term saffron consumption improves retinal flicker sensitivity in early age-related macular degeneration beyond its antioxidant activity. (37)

Preparation: Measured dietary supplement 1 mg extract/kg/d or 100 mg/kg po.

Caution: Side effects from the consumption of saffron are midland consist of dizziness, nausea, drowsiness, appetite increase or suppression, anxiety, and the occasional allergic reaction of rash, hives, and mucous membrane swelling.

Broccoli, cabbage, corn, pepper, and spinach, by virtue of their high content of the macular pigments, lutein, and zeaxanthin, are associated with a lower risk of age-related macular degeneration. A pilot study of four groups with and without drusen and neovascularization and eating five portions or less of fruit and vegetables per day was conducted. An analysis of the mean optical density measured by the MPS 9000 QuantifEYE, confirmed the positive impact of food supplementation on the optical density. (38) The intake of broccoli prevented cataractogenesis in albino rats through its antioxidant activity and ionic balance trough the Ca(2+) ATPase pump, inhibition of lipid peroxidation, calpain activation, and protein insolubilization. (39)

Preparation: Cooked: steamed, boiled, fried in oil...as desired.

Caution: Green and red peppers are plants of the nightshade family, containing nitrogen-based alkaloids, which may be toxic when consumed raw in moderate to large quantities. Young plants have a higher content of toxic chemicals. Cooking reduces toxicity.

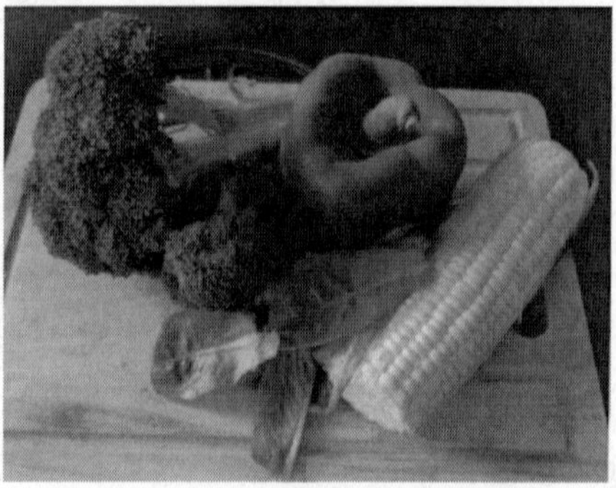

Figure 1. Antioxidant Vegetables

Conventional treatments for blepharitis and conjunctivitis depend on the etiology as being bacterial, allergic, viral, fungal, ocular surface disease from deficiency or excess, or trauma. They consist of hygiene, topical pharmaceutical-based antibiotics, steroids, antihistaminics, antifungals, and tear film substitutes. Viral infections are aggressively treated with acyclovir or trifluridines with support from lubricants and decongestants. Bacterial infections are treated with third and fourth generation fluoroquinolones and resistant strains are still developing. Allergy shots over several months may work to reduce sensitivity to an allergen, but results are variable. Antihistamine eyedrops consisting mainly of a vasoconstrictor with antazoline or olopatadine, sting in an already compromised inflamed eye eliciting patient complaints and possible noncompliance. In many cases, the application of cool compresses work best through natural vasoconstriction.

Caution: Severe and persistent red eyes with pain and discharge require medical care.

Eyebright	Calendula	Goldenseal	Borage oil
Chamomile	Aloe vera	Spanish needle	Witch hazel
Yarrow	Honeysuckle	Flaxseed	Chrysanthemum

Table 3. Botanicals for Eye infection/inflammation *
(*Best used as compresses applied to eyelids or
as topical eyedrops; all evidence-based)

Eyebright (*Euphrasia offinialis*) is an anti-inflammatory herb with pyrrolizidine alkaloids, iridoid glycosides, tannins, resins, mannite, glucose, acrid bitter principle, volatile oil, and euphrasia-tannin acid. It relieves inflammation of the eyes and mucous membranes caused by colds, sinus infections, chemical irritants, and allergies. It has strong astringent activity, which reduces copious secretions and also causes vasoconstriction to staunch bleeding from minor abrasions. (40) (41)

Preparation: External eyewash; 1 ounce (4–6 leaves), chopped, steeped in hot water, cooled and instilled with an eyedropper 2–3 times daily; may be applied as a poultice; or taken internally as a tea for relief of general inflammation.

Caution: Pyrrrolizidine alkaloids can be toxic to liver, so consumption as a tea should be limited. The efficacy and safety of eyebright has not been proven by the FDA.

Calendula (*C. offinialis*) also known as marigold, is primarily used for treating skin abrasions and wounds and can be used for wound healing of lid lacerations and postoperative lid procedures (41). When combined with acyclovir, it accelerates the resolution of herpetic keratitis. (42) Its anti-inflammatory activity is effective in the treatment of blepharitis and conjunctivitis. (43) (44) Its medicinal actions are due to triterpenoid compounds such as oleanolic acid which inhibit bacterial activity and antioxidant effect, which reduces damage done by free radicals. It has both a detergent and a vulnerary effect on wounds.

Preparation: As an eyewash, cream or compress for dry skin (eczematous lids) wound healing, sore eyes and as a tincture, two drops in one cup hot water, cool and apply twice daily.

Goldenseal (*Hydrastis Canadensis*) is an anti-inflammatory herb with alkaloids (berberine, hydrastine and palmitine), which exhibit a beneficial effect on bacterial eye infections and inflammations, acute pterygium, and viral and allergic conjunctivitis. (45) It acts as an antiseptic, detergent, astringent, antibiotic, and alterative particularly on mucous membranes.

Preparation: The roots are mashed into a powder, boiled in water, cooled and applied to the eye with an eyecup; it may be combined with boric water as an eyebath. Works well when combined with eyebright.

Caution: Eating the fresh plant can cause inflammation of the mucous tissues and possible ulcerations. Eyewashes containing berberine may cause phototoxicity when the eyes are exposed to bright sunlight.

Borage (*B.officinalis*), when supplemented in the diet with GLA (gamma-linolenic acid) oils has proven consistently superior to EPA in the reduction of neovascular responses and chronic inflammation as a result of alkali burn to the eyes of rabbits to reduce severity of structural damage. (46) It contains high amounts of potassium and calcium for fluid regulation and mineral acids and common salts for demulcent, emollient, and refrigerant effects on inflamed mucous membranes.

Preparation: The leaves are steeped as a tea, cooled, and applied as a compress for tired inflamed eyes.

Caution: Contact with fresh leaves may cause dermatitis in sensitive individuals.

Chamomile (*Matricaria recutita*) contains bitter extractive, tannic acid, and volatile oils, which promote tissue regeneration through granulation when applied to eyelid inflammation caused by the parasite, Demodex folliculorum. (47) It has been used traditionally for healing traumatic eyelid wounds.

Preparation: It is as commercially available as Cepan cream, a combination of onion extract, heparin, and chamomile extract allantoin. Boiled water may be added to the dried flowers, and the warm extract applied to eyelids as tolerated.

Caution: A hypersensitive reaction in the conjunctival and corneal tissues, and/or contact dermatitis to lids may occur in certain susceptible individuals from the use of compresses.

Spanish needle (*Bidens pilosa*) contains polyacetylenes with phenylheptatriyne, which are activated by daylight and along with linolic and linoleic acids, have antimicrobial activity. (48) Water and alcohol extracts contain prostaglandin-synthesis inhibitors and the flavonoids, friedlain and friedlan-3 beta-ol, which exhibit strong anti-inflammatory activity by inhibiting COX-1 and -2 enzymes. (49)

Preparation: Fresh juice from the leaves may be squeezed directly into eyes.

There are no known or documented side effects or contraindications.

Witch hazel (*Hamamelis virginiana*) acts predominantly as an astringent and antimicrobial. It contains tannin, gallic acid, catechins, proanthrocyanins, flavonoids, essential oils, choline, and saponins, which are especially effective in the relief of symptoms and repair of lid abrasions, injuries with hematoma and eczematous dermatitis. It is used in children as a first line since safety and efficacy are rated as excellent. (50)

Preparation: Boiling the leaves, bark and stems of the shrub produces a distillate on condensation, which is used as a compress. Commercial witch hazel is readily available.

Caution: Large doses taken by mouth may cause liver problems. It may cause minor skin irritation in some people.

Yarrow (*Achillea millefolium*) is a strong astringent, which has been used traditionally for hemostasis of wounds, cuts, and abrasions. Since it contains tannins, asparagin, sterols, salicylic acid, flavonoids, isovaleric acid, and coumarins, it has been said to both stop bleeding and promote it. It has been used effectively in rejuvenation of the eyelid skin (reducing wrinkles and opening pores) in the cosmetic industry. (51)

Preparation: The essential oil is extracted by steam distillation of the flowers and applied directly to the affected surface.

Caution: In rare cases, yarrow can cause a severe allergic skin rash and prolonged use may increase photosensitivity in the skin. (52)

Honeysuckle (*Lonicera caerulea*) contains the phenolics, cyanidin3-glucoside, cyaniding 3-rutinoside, and chlorogenic acid and is used primarily in medicinal cough syrups. Blue honeysuckle extract (BHE) had a positive inflammation attenuating effect on endotoxin-induced uveitis in rats by inhibiting the production of proinflammatory mediators in the COX-2 pathway. (53)

Preparation: An extract of flowers and leaves can be distilled, collected, cooled, and applied directly to the eyes.

Caution: Though characterized by the sweet odor of its flowers, the berries can be mildly poisonous.

Flaxseed (*Linum usitatissimam*) oil contains high levels of the omega-3 compound, alpha-linolenic acid (ALA), which is converted into two different fatty acids, eicosapentaenoic acid (EPA) and docosahexaenoic acid (DHA), which protect cell membranes. There was a 70 percent improvement in symptoms and signs in a pilot, prospective, randomized, double-masked, placebo-controlled clinical trial in the average tear production and tear volume in patients with symptomatic dry eyes. The recommended dietary supplementation includes fish oil, 450 mg EPA, 300 mg DHA, and 1000 mg flaxseed oil. In another study, flaxseed oil capsules at a dosage of 1 or 2 grams per day also reduced the symptoms of ocular surface inflammation and dry eye in Sjogren's syndrome patients. (54) (55) A possible mechanism of action involves the reduction of inflammation by directly generating anti-inflammatoory prostaglandins (prostaglandin E3 and leukotriene B5), blocking the gene expression of the proinflammatory cytokines, tumor necrosis factor alpha and interleukin-1 alpha and interleukin-1 beta, working synergistically with fish oil to inhibit omega-6, which results in reduction of arachidonic acid. (56)

Preparation: Ground flaxseed 1–2 teaspoons daily with cereal or food or by itself, or 1–2 grams per day in capsule or liquid form are suggested.

Caution: Both flaxseed oil and fish oil can increase the risk of bleeding if one is taking conventional blood thinners. Notifying and discussing supplementation with a medical professional is recommended.

Chrysanthemum (*C. indicum*) contains flavanone glycosides, which were shown to inhibit the enzyme, aldose reductase, that catalyses cataract formation in diabetes and galactosemia in the rat lens. (57) When used with artificial tears, it was found to alleviate dry eye symptoms, prolong tear break up time (TBUT) and promote the secretion of tears in postmenopausal women with xerophthalmia. (58) It is included in the herbal beverage remedy for *Hot Qi* allergies in children in Hong Kong, for its ability to soothe itchy eyes. (59) It reduces the capillary permeability induced by histamine when taken internally. In addition to the active glycosides, it contains alkaloids, the essential oil, bornol, and flavonoids, luteolin and apigenin.

Preparation: The flower parts are steeped into a tea and consumed 1–2 times daily. It may be cooled and used as a compress over the eyes.

There were no reported side effects from its usage.

Willow bark	Ginger	Turmeric	Boswellia

Table 4. Botanicals for Eye Pain:

Eye pain may result from serious conditions such as angle-closure glaucoma and infections like cellulitis and endophthalmitis, which are not amenable to herbal treatments. Eye pain associated with the inflammation of colds and flu, arthritis and trauma may benefit from the following herbal remedies. For those individuals who are susceptible to side effects of conventional painkillers, such as ulcers, decreased white blood cell count, intestinal bleeding, and liver damage, as well as to the addictive properties of opioids, the natural herbal anti-inflammatories are a viable choice for pain relief. Their mechanism of action involves reduction of inflammation and swelling in the tissues in and around the eye, without the side effects.

Caution: Severe or persistent eye pain requires immediate medical care.

Willow bark (*Salix alba*) contains salicin, which is the prodrug metabolized during absorption into the various salicylate derivatives. Flavonoids and polyphenols contribute to the characteristic analgesic and anti-inflammatory effect. This multicomponent activity provides a broader mechanism of action than commercial aspirin and without the serious side effects of gastrointestinal mucosal damage and blood thinning. (60)

Preparation: The salicylic acid is concentrated more heavily in the sap. Steep one teaspoon of standardized willow bark in one cup of hot water, strain and drink one to three cups per day.

Caution: May be associated with allergic skin reactions. Like aspirin, it should be avoided in pregnancy or breastfeeding, and in children with fever, to avoid the possibility of Reye's Syndrome. People on blood thinners should be aware of the dosage, though it has less of an effect than aspirin.

Ginger (*Zingiber officinale*) contains gingerols, which inhibit the production of nitric oxide, a major component in the pathway of inflammatory hyperalgesia. (61) It is especially appropriate for mild to moderate swelling around the eyes associated with arthritis, aging, and lack of rest. In addition, it improves blood circulation in peripheral vessels and has some antiviral properties. (62)

Preparation: The average dose of ginger root capsules can range from 100–1000 mg, and can be taken as powder or tea. Fresh ginger can be sliced, diced, minced, and added to food and soups. Commercial extracts are available.

Caution: Has an additive blood thinning effect when used with warfarin or coumarin. It should be avoided in gallbladder disease as it promotes bile production. Overdose can lead to symptoms of anxiety.

Turmeric (*Curcuma longa*) is closely related to ginger and also has strong anti-inflammatory properties with antioxidant, tissue-healing properties, and pain-reducing effects. The active ingredient is curcumin, a natural phenol, which exhibits its effects by inhibiting COX-2 enzymes in the inflammatory pathway to eicosanoid biosynthesis, lipid peroxidation, and oxidative DNA damage. It was found to be effective in reducing inflammatory eye disease and postoperative pain. (63)

Preparation: Available in powder form to add to food or make a tea, capsules at a recommended dosage of two to three grams daily, and standardized extract of curcumin. Adding black pepper increases absorption.

Caution: High doses cause relatively few side effects, with some reporting mild nausea and diarrhea. (64) It was found to alter iron metabolism causing iron deficiency in certain susceptible patients. (65)

Boswellia (*B. serrata*) is an Indian frankincense herb used most effectively for reducing inflammation in rheumatoid and osteoarthritis. The active principles are boswellic acids isolated from the gum resin of *Boswellia serrata*, which inhibited the leukotriene synthesis via 5-lipoxygenase from arachidonic acid. (66) (67) (68) It is useful for reducing swelling and pain around the eye.

Preparation: Available in its natural form as a gum resin and as a cream, sometimes with capsaicin and methyl salicylate for added pain relief.

Boswellia gum oleresin has been applied directly to eye tissues with only minor irritation and no long-term side effects.

Cataract

Cineraria maritima	Tulsi	Fenugreek
Green tea	Turmeric	Ginger
Mormordica charantia	*Bilberry*	*Grapeseed extract*

Table 5. Botanicals for Specific eye conditions:

In experimental models, selenite-induced cataractogenesis was mediated by oxidative stress, which led to the accumulation of calcium and activation of lenticular calpains, a super family of Ca2+ dependent proteases, which are involved in proteolysis and insolubilization of lens protein. Substances that can reduce stress-induced protein oxidation, deactivate the calpains, inhibit the Ca2+ ATPase, and prevent the accumulation of calcium, would be effective in protecting the lens from cataract formation. (70) An ethanolic extract of *Cineraria maritima* (*C. maritima*) was found to prevent selenite-induced cataractogenesis both in vitro and in vivo, by modulating the activity of the antioxidant enzymes, catalase, gluthathione peroxidase, and superoxide dismutase. Homeopathic cineraria is available in generic and as cataract care for use topically two to three times a day. No side effects have been reported.

An aqueous extract of the Ayurvedic herb, tulsi (*Ocimum sanctum*), showed anticataractogenic activity against selenite-induced experimental cataractogenesis by restoration of the antioxidant defense system and inhibition of protein insolubilization in rat lenses. The effective dose was 5–10 mg/kg in reducing the incidence of cataract by 20 percent and 60 percent respectively.

Fenugreek (*Trigonella foenum-graecum*) prevented cataractogenesis in vitro and in vivo in rat lenses by maintaining glutathione levels and reducing malonialdehyde levels via significant restoration of the antioxidant enzymes, glutathione peroxidase, superoxide dismutase, catalase, and glutathione-S-transferase. The significance warrants human trials.

By virtue of the modulation of biochemical parameters by its polyphenolic compounds, green tea (*Camillia sinensis*) was found to prevent selenite-induced cataractogenesis by preserving the antioxidant defense system. Epigallocatechin gallate, the main component, protects the human lens epithelial cells from mitochondria-mediated apoptosis induced by peroxidation, through its regulation of caspase enzymes and the MAPK and Akt pathways.

Turmeric (*Curcuma longa*) reduced free radical-mediated cataractogenesis through its prevention of accumulation of calcium in the lens. At a dose of 75 mg/kg body weight, it was shown to activate Ca2+ ATPase and inhibit lens opacification in rat pups. The significant results supports the possibility that the natural consumption of curcumin in food may help prevent the onset of senile cataracts in the human lens.

In streptozotocin-induced diabetic cataracts, ginger (*Zingiber officinalis*) was effective against the development of lens opacification through its antiglycolating potential and its inhibition of the polyol pathway. Incorporating ginger in the diet may be explored for the prevention of diabetic cataracts.

A lysophilized aqueous extract of the Afro-Asian vine, *Momordica charantia*, was given orally to alloxan-treated rats, and found to prevent the development of cataract, along with significant reduction in plasma glucose levels in one group and delay the development of cataract in another group. Also known as bitter melon and maidenapple, its active constituents are mormordicin and cucurbitacin B, which hae insulin-like activity. It also contains terpenoids, glycosides, and cytotoxic proteins, which deactivate ribosomes. The bitter-tasting seeds contain vicine, which can trigger symptoms of favism in susceptible individuals. The red arils are toxic to children. Eating the fruit is contraindicated in pregnancy.

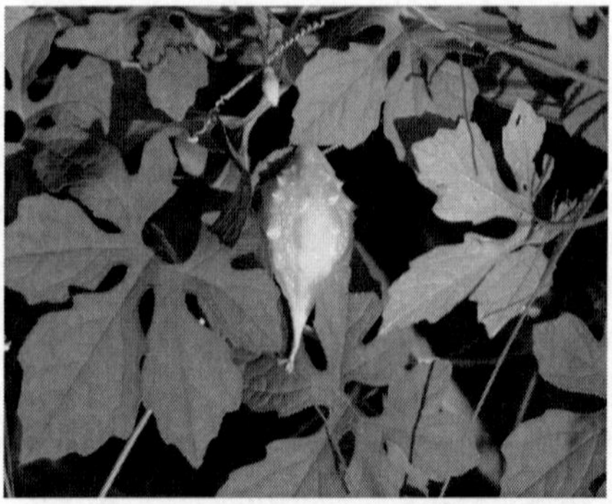

Figure 2. *Momordica charantia*

Glaucoma

Marijuana	Fennel seeds	Forskolin
Sage	Bael fruit	Ginkgo biloba

Table 6.

The prevention and treatment of glaucomatous optic neuropathy is based on the lowering of intraocular pressure through regulation of aqueous inflow and outflow dynamics and blood flow to the optic nerve head.

In November of 1979, clinical researchers at Howard University Hospital (Washington, DC), first reported that the inhalation of marijuana (*Cannabis sativa*), containing 2.8 percent delta-9-tetrahydrocannabinol, reduced both the intraocular pressure (IOP) of eyes with glaucoma and blood pressure, both most likely due to the effects of its peripheral vasodilatory properties. (81) Psychophysiological side effects of increased heart rate, blood pressure, and altered mentality may not be conducive to its routine use as an efficient antiglaucoma medication. With the expansion of clinical trials, the IOP decreased post inhalation, heart rate increased, and blood pressure decreased. The decreases in systolic and diastolic blood pressures were greater in hypertensive glaucoma subjects than in normotensive glaucoma subjects. (82) (83)

Topical administration, though effective in laboratory animals, was not shown to be effective in humans with primary open-angle glaucoma at the doses of 0.05 and 0.1 percent. (84) The most serious side effect was orthostatic hypotension characterized by sudden bradycardia (HR<50/min), light-headedness, and fainting. This complex was observed in a long-term marijuana user as well as in naïve marijuana users. There was no correlation of orthostatic hypotension with either blood plasma levels of delta 9-THC or previous marijuana experience. (85) The oral administration of delta 9-THC was used in nonsmokers or in those individuals in whom inhalation was difficult. There were seven subjects with glaucoma that experienced a decrease in IOP though the accompanying side effects (dysphoria, depersonalization/anxiety, and paranoid-like reactions) were frequent; hence these adverse effects were reported to the NIDA and future studies involved lower dosages with 5, 10 mg, or placebo capsules. In ten glaucoma subjects unable to smoke marijuana, all three dosages seemed to lower the IOP at four to six hours. Heart rate increased by 11.4+/-2.6 beats per minute and the systolic blood pressure decreased 8.6+/2.4 mmHg at one hour. One marijuana-naïve subject experienced orthostatic hypotension after only 5 mg oral delta 9-THC. Future clinical trials with either inhaled marijuana or oral cannabinoids were no longer performed after 1982 due to changes in governmental policies. (86) Modern medicine needs to reinstitute active research into the ability of cannabis to relieve pain and reduce symptoms of some neurodegenerative and arthritic diseases, the nausea and vomiting of chemotherapy, and the intraocular pressure of glaucoma.

Fennel seeds (*Foeniculum vulgare*) contain anethole as the active ingredient. The aqueous seed extract demonstrated significant ocular hypotensive activity, which was found to be comparable to that of timolol maleate 0.5 percent. Fennel seeds can be eaten raw or the leaves can be consumed as vegetables or cooked as part of a meal. As an anise-flavored spice, it is used in culinary recipes worldwide. Aside from hypersensitivity, it is generally well-tolerated. (88)

Derived from the leaves of the African coleus plant, topical *forskolin*, a naturally occurring diterpene, lowered the intraocular pressure in human subjects with primary open-angle glaucoma by reducing aqueous inflow through stimulation of adenylate cyclase activity. Outflow facility remained unchanged and ciliary blood flow increased through its vasorelaxant effect. (89) (90) The oral administration of forskolin, along with rutin and vitamins B1 and B2, also demonstrated an additional reduction in intraocular pressure. (91)

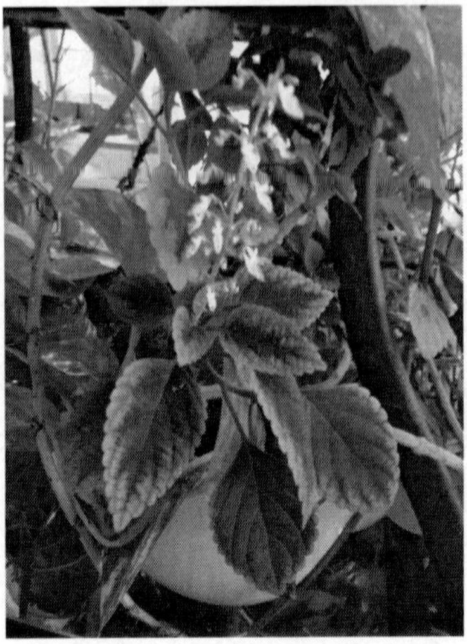

Figure 3. *Coleus forskohlii*

The intramuscular injection of an extract of *sage* (*Salvia miltiorrhiza*) has been shown to improve visual acuity and peripheral vision on people with glaucoma, through its action on retrograde axoplasmic transport in improving the microcirculation of the retinal ganglion cells and tolerance of the nerve tissue to anoxia. (92) (93) Intravenous administration of *Salvia miltiorrhiza* in rabbits significantly demonstrated optic nerve protection when compared to those treated with saline. Neither group showed reduction in intraocular pressure nor were there significant side effects. (94)

The pulp of the bael fruit (*Aegle marmelos*) contains phenolics, alkaloids, terpenoids, flavonoids, glutathione reductase and peroxidase, catalases, glutamate transaminases, and many other antioxidants, which inhibit lipid peroxidation and glutamine metabolism. The aqueous extract of the fruit at a dosage of 0.15 was applied topically to water-loaded and steroid-induced rabbit eyes. Its IOP lowering effect compared favorably to that of 0.25 percent timolol maleate. In rabbits with normal IOP, it showed a 22.8 percent reduction from baseline. The exact mechanism is unknown. (95) (96)

Ginkgo biloba lowered intraocular pressure through its antioxidant properties and its effects on increasing blood flow in small vessels. By deactivation binding of free radicals, the enzyme GCLC directly scavenged O2 and OH and inhibited lipid peroxidation. The extract of ginkgo exhibited stronger antioxidant activity than flavonoids and terpenoids. (97) The increase in blood flow may directly benefit the optic nerve in preventing and improving glaucomatous optic neuropathy. (98) Oral *Ginkgo biloba* extract at a dosage of 40 mg three times a day, appeared to improve preexisting visual field damage in some patients with normal tension glaucoma. (99) The IOP-lowering effect of ginkgo is too small for it to be used routinely in the current management of glaucoma. In one study, the topical application of an extract of ginkgo exerted a therapeutic effect on the treatment of seasonal allergic conjunctivitis. (100)

Preparation: Ginkgo biloba is available as a tea to be taken two to three cups daily or in capsules and extract at an average dosage of 60–120 mg per day. Tincture of three to five ml drops in a cup of water may also be used.

Caution: Use of *Ginkgo biloba* has been linked to spontaneous hyphema due to its blood thinning properties. It has been associated with the precipitation of seizures in epilepsy patients. (101)

Diabetes

Bitter melon	Cinnamon bark	*Tulsi*	Stevia
Gymnema	Aloe vera	Ginseng	Ashwagandha
Garlic	Green tea	Noni	Psyllium

Table 7

The treatment of eye diseases associated with hyperglycemia with botanicals is based on the fact that lowering blood glucose levels results in a reduced incidence and prevalence of pathology. As there are too many botanicals with hypoglycemic effects to include in this chapter, the following are some of the more common.

Bitter melon (*Mormordica charantia*) has both hypoglycemic and hypotensive activity. Cucurbitane triterpenoids activate the enzyme AMPK, a protein that regulates glucose uptake. Other compounds, vicine and charantin, increase fatty acid oxidation and increase glucose disposal in the body. Significant amounts of vitamin C, fiber, B vitamins, magnesium, potassium, and zinc also contribute. (102) Oral administrations of a whole-plant aqueous extract was used on normal and diabetic rats with chlorpropamide as a reference resulted in significant hypoglycemia. (103) A randomized clinical trial conducted on forty patients found a decline in A1c of 1 percent at the outset, but was unable to make a definite conclusion. (104) Another study found no conclusive evidence compared with placebo. (105) Alcohol and aqueous extracts of *Momordica charantia* administered at three varying doses of 50, 100, 200 mg/kg/day produced a mean reduction in plasma glucose levels of 15 to 22 percent. (106) At best, the hypoglycemic effect is moderate.

Preparation: Oral aqueous extract of leaves and fruit at a dosage of 100–200 mg/kg/day.

Caution: Possible hypoglycemic coma and convulsions in children, headaches and favism-like syndrome. It may have additive effects when taken with other hypoglycemics. (107)

Cinnamon bark (*Cinnamomum burmannii*) extract contains the polyphenol compound, methylhydroxychalcone, which stimulates the insulin receptors in the formation of glycogen. By inhibiting alpha-glucosidase, it effectively suppresses postprandial hyperglycemia. Since it has no effect on A1C, fasting blood glucose, lipid metabolism, or type 1 diabetes, it is not a suitable replacement for conventional hypoglycemics. However, it may be used as an adjunctive supplement. (108) (109) (110)

Preparation: Available in capsules a daily dosage of one to six grams; one to two-inch stick may be steeped in a tea and taken two to three times a day; or as a powder in a drink or on food, one teaspoon daily.

Caution: As a diaphoretic, it may lead to increased detoxification when added to licorice and ginger. It has blood-thinning properties and may lead to liver toxicity when taken in large doses over a long period of time. It is not recommended during pregnancy.

The bioactive component of the tulsi (*Ocimum sanctum*) plant is in its aerial parts and consists of a tetracyclic triterpenoid, which exibits potent antidiabetic activity by reducing glucose, as well as total cholesterol and triglycerides. (111) Also known as *Holy basil*, it is an adaptogen which promotes a sense of well-being and provides relief from symptoms of common cold, flu, and stress-related maladies by strengthening the immune system.

Preparation. One cup of tea daily is preventive and two to three cups in times of illness is recommended.

Caution: Overdosing may lead to hypotension and hypersensitivity reactions.

Known as a natural sweetener, stevia (*S. rebaudiana*) extract from the leaves was found to have a revitalizing effect on beta cells of the pancreas. The active ingredients are steviol glycosides, which only cause a mild decrease in blood glucose level and may even enhance glucose tolerance. (112) It was shown to increase insulin sensitivity in rats and possibly promote insulin production. (113)

Preparation: Available in capsules, liquid, or powder. Experimental dosage was 200–400 mg/kg.

Caution: Aside from the occasional reports of bloating, nausea, and dizziness, there are no confirmed adverse effects for humans.

The extract of gymnema (*G. sylvestre*) contains gymnemic acids, a group of oleanane-type triterpenoid saponins, glycosides, and alkaloids, which have antidiabetic, antisweetener, and anti-inflammatory activities. In addition to increasing circulating insulin and reducing both fasting and postprandial blood sugar levels, the herb also reduced the taste of sugar in the mouth by blocking the taste receptors on the tongue, thereby controlling cravings. (114) (115)

Preparation: Available as standardized capsules of 250 mg leaf and 75 percent gymnemic acids, tid with meals or as extract 520 mg capsules.

Caution: Reported side effects are few except for one case of toxic hepatitis with long-term use. (116)

An alcoholic extract of *Aloe vera* leaf gel significantly decreased blood glucose levels and reversed elevated lipid peroxidation and hydroperoxides in tissues of diabetic rats. This was accompanied by an increase in reduced glutathione, superoxide dismutase, catalase, glutathione peroxidase, and glutathione-S-transmutase in the liver and kidney, thereby showing strong antioxidant activity. (117) The positive effects of antioxidant free radical scavenging relating to the prevention and treatment of diabetes are well documented. (118)

Preparation: A leaf gel extract is available commercially as a juice. Aloe gel can be diluted 50 percent with an unsweetened fruit juice and taken two to three times daily as a tonic, immune system booster, purgative, digestive and blood sugar regulator.

Caution: Mild stomach pain and nausea may occur.

Both the root and the berry of *Panax ginseng* have displayed significant hypoglycemic activity. In addition, the berry-reduced body weight in experimental diabetic rats. (119) In another study, ginsenoside Rh2 in the *Panax ginseng* root, improved insulin sensitivity and was suggested as being suitable for use as an adjuvant for diabetic patients. (120)

In a human study, neither ginseng nor its active component, ginsenoside Re, improved the beta-cell function or reduced body weight in patients with diabetes. Lack of adequate bioavailability may have been the cause of reduced therapeutic effect. (121)

Preparation: Available as standardized extract 100–200 mg daily; powdered form or capsules of 500–1000 mg for tea or oral administration; the root may be simmered in hot water for forty-five to sixsty minutes for several cups a day.

Caution: Additive effect in lowering the blood sugar in diabetics on conventional medications; some nausea, anxiety, stomach upset, and insomnia may occur.

Ashwagandha root (*Withania somnifera*) and leaf extracts contain phenolic compounds and flavonoids, which exert strong antioxidant activity in lowering blood glucose levels in diabetic rats.

Also known as *Indian ginseng*, its active ingredients are alkaloids, of which withanine is the main constituent, and steroidal lactones, consisting of withanolides. (122)

Preparation: Decoct one teaspoon of root powder in one cup of hot water.

Caution: It is a member of the nightshade family and has hepatotoxic effects when taken in excess.

Garlic (*Allium sativum*) reduced blood glucose by improving insulin sensitivity in experimentally controlled diabetic rats. It also reduced triglyceride and uric acid levels, and normalized nitric oxide levels. There was also a positive effect in reduction of body weight and serum glycated hemoglobin; thereby, showing attenuation of metabolic syndrome and oxidative stress. (123)

Preparation: Raw garlic clove, dried powder extract, tablets or capsules 600–900 mg taken daily could benefit diabetic health.

Aside from socially unacceptable breath, garlic has few serious side effects. Its blood-thinning activity on platelets may be additive, so it is practical to discontinue use before surgery.

Green tea (*Camillia sinensis*) supplementation reduced insulin-stimulated glucose uptake, insulin binding of adipocytes and glucose transporter IV content of adipocytes in fructose-fed laboratory animals. In addition to their many beneficial healthy activities, the epigallocatechins in green tea are effective in the regulation of diabetic glucose levels. (124)

Preparation: Steep one teaspoon of leaves in hot water for tea that may be taken two to three times daily. Available as capsules 500 mg daily.

Caution: Excessive use has been associated with hepatotoxicity.

Diabetic rats were treated with fermented noni (*Morinda citrifolia*) juice (2 ml/kg twice a day) and compared with a reference drug, glibenciamide. Both groups showed significant reduction in blood glucose levels, as well as improvement in fatty degeneration of their livers. (125) It contains the active phytochemicals, scopoletin and damnacanthal.

Preparation: Fermented extract and juice from the fruit of the tree must be thoroughly boiled and hydraulically pressed and re-boiled to separate the drink from the pulp and to remove the toxins containing anthraquinones. Available as organic pasteurized or unpasteurized products.

Caution: Excess use can lead to extreme hypoglycemia, hyperkalemia affecting the kidneys, acute hepatitis, skin eruptions, respiratory difficulties, and digestion irregularities.

The addition of psyllium (*Plantago ovate*), with significant fiber and mucilage, to the diabetic diet was shown to improve gastric tolerance to the conventional hypoglycemic, metformin. Both fasting blood glucose levels and HbA1c showed significant reduction. There were no adverse effects. (126)

Preparation. Mix one to two teaspoons of powder in water and drink twice daily before meals.

Caution: Psyllium can reduce the absorption of certain other drugs, like digoxin, so should not be taken together. Should be avoided in patients with a history of gastrointestinal obstruction or previous bowel surgery.

**Italicized botanicals discussed in Table 1.*

Tea	Passionflower	Cassia seed	Amla	Atractylodes	Prunella
Eyewash	Fennel	Wild okra	Aloe vera	Elder flowers	Cortadura b.
Compress	Bastard okra	Burdock root	Forsynthia	Goldenseal	Prickly pear
Red rasp	Vervain	Hog plum	Llantén	Rosewater	Chickweed

Table 8. Traditional herbal medicine for eyes around the world**

Due to the active ingredients of botanicals, daily dosages have been advocated for swollen eyelids, red, itchy eyes, vision enhancement, and even glaucoma. Many of the treatments have not been through clinical trials and do not have evidence-based western approval. It is not possible to account for all the botanicals used for eye treatment in the world, but the following are some of the more common botanicals used for which there is little or no scientific evidence in the literature. There is a solid case, based on age-long success, as well as economic grounds, for integrating traditional medicines into modern eye care systems.

**Not evidence based

Passionflower (*Passiflora incarnata*) has been found to improve small-vessel blood flow and act on brain enzymes at same sites as GABA neurotransmitter to induce drowsiness for insomnia. It is purported to prevent glaucomatous optic neuropathy.

Cassia (cinnamon) seed (Jue Ming Zi) can be taken as a tea for dry, swollen, red, painful eyes. It has been most often used in a mixture with *Chrysanthemum* flowers.

Aamla (Indian gooseberry) is an Ayurvedic herbal antioxidant with high levels of vitamin C recommended for treating eye infections.

Atractylodes (*A. rhizoma*) (Cang Zhu) is an herb that has been used for thousands of years in Chinese medicine for treating night blindness and general eye health. It has high levels of vitamin A.

Xia Ku Cao, (*Spica prunellae*) herb has been used mainly for reducing nodules as well as for swollen, red, painful eyes by reducing liver inflammation.

Fennel seeds and roots (*Foeniculum vulgare)* have been bruised and added to boiled water and used as an eyewash to detoxify and treat infection, ease tired, dry eyes, and clear cloudy vision. It must be made fresh daily.

Wild okra, *Malachra alceaefolia*, fruit can be macerated and the juice used as an eyewash for inflamed noninfective conjunctivitis.

Aloe vera has shown significant activity for wound healing for thermal burns and periorbital abrasions. The fresh gel is diluted to 50 percent in boiled water, cooled, and applied directly to skin wounds or to corneal lacerations for enhanced healing. Antimicrobial activity precludes sterility as the observed results are positive. It should be mixed fresh every three days for maximum effect and safety.

Elder flowers can be steeped, cooled, and applied with an eyedropper for tired eyes.

Cortadora Blanca, *Scleria pterota*, is boiled and cooled, and applied to active pterygium eyes for reduction in size and inflammation.

Bastard Okra, *Melachra alceifolia*, leaves are boiled and strained. The liquid is applied in a compress to soothe burning, inflamed eyes.

Burdock root *(Arctium lappa)* is a blood purifier, liver tonic, and lymphatic cleanser, which can be used as compresses for styes.

Forsythia (*F. suspensa*) is a cooling herb with antiviral and antibacterial activities, which can be used for eye infections.

Goldenseal (*Hydrastis canadensis*) is well-known for its antibacterial and antiseptic properties. It can be used as a compress to treat eye inflammation.

Prickly pear (*Opuntia dillenii*) can be crushed and the juice mixed with water and used as a cool compress for inflamed eyes. It contains alkaloids, which act on the inflammation pathway to reduce the hypersensitive reaction.

Red raspberry leaf (*Rubus idaeus*) is an astringent herb that may remove excess mucous from the eyes.

Vervain (*Verbena officinalis*) leaves can be boiled in water and used as a hot compress for eye inflammation.

Hog plum (*Spondias mombin*) can be used as a compress for inflamed eyes by placing buds, roots and bark into boiled water.

Llantén (*Plantago major*) contains the iroid glycoside, aucubin, a powerful coagulant and allantoin, a cell proliferant. A decoction of leaves when cooled, may be applied to traumatized eyelids to reduce bleeding and aid in the resolution of a hematoma.

Rosewater compresses can be made from the distillate of rose petals and used for soothing tired, burning, red eyes with dark circles.

Chickweed (*Stellaria media*), has high levels of vitamin C, calcium, magnesium and potassium, and is used to reduce eyelid swelling.

Wolfberry flowers, goji berry, triphala, *Chrysanthemum*, lyceum, mulberry, and stinkingweed (*Cassia occidentalis*) are all used in traditional medicine to prevent and reduce cataracts as well as to prevent and treat retino-macular degenerations.

The average frequency of tea consumption is twice a day. Eyewash is recommended for three to four times a day. Compresses may be applied for twenty minutes every hour for three to four hours until relieved. Note that if not properly prepared, the eyewash and compresses may introduce bacteria into the eye.

Contact

Blinding tree	Manchineel	Oleander	Dieffenbachia
Prickly pear	Cashew nut tree	Poinsettia	Croton
Acalypha	Philodendron	Calla lily	Anthurium
Squirting cucumber	Chamomile	Stinging spurge	Ortiga

Table 9. Ocular side effects of Botanicals:

The defense mechanisms of certain plants involve the mechanical release of chemical agents such as steroidal glycosides, atropine, and alkaloid teratogens, which may cause symptoms, which range from irritation to irreversible damage to the cornea and conjunctiva upon contact. The most common symptoms include eyelid edema, conjunctival hyperemia, corneal edema and clouding, itching, blurred vision, and disturbances in color vision. Severe keratoconjunctivitis may occur from contact with the sap of blinding tree, manchineel, oleander, dieffenbachia, and prickly pear. (127) Exposure of the ocular tissues to the undiluted juice of the squirting cucumber (*Ecbalium elaterium*) led to immediate conjunctivitis and corneal edema. (128) The flowers of cashew nut tree, chamomile and poinsettia, and the leaves of croton, acalypha, philodendron, calla, anthurium, stinging spurge, and ortiga give a milder irritation to eye tissues. Plants that cause conjunctivitis by virtue of their release of pollen include trees (hickory, poplar, sycamore, and maple), grasses (Bermuda, timothy, orchard, and sweet vernal), and flowering weeds with powdery granules. Molds (*Eurotium*), fungi (*Fusarium*), and yeast (*Candida*) may also cause severe keratitis.

Ingestion

Mushroom	Soursop	Datura	Licorice	Oleander
Dieffenbachia	Jimson weed	Angels trumpet	St johns wort	A.belladonna

Table 10. Ocular side effects of Botanicals

Plants of the nightshade (*Atropa belladonna*), dogbane (*Nerium oleander*) and Solanaceae (*Brugmansia suaveolens*) families, and Datura species (Jimson weed) contain anticholinergic alkaloids, which can cause mydriasis and angle-closure glaucoma in susceptible eyes. Ingestion of mushrooms (*Cantharellus cinnabarinus*) containing the carotenoid, canthaxanthin, can cause abnormal ERG, static threshold perimetry, changes in dark adaptaion, and crystalline retinopathy. (129) Overconsumption of soursop (*Annona muricata*), also known as graviola, which is touted for its anticancer activity, can lead to an atypical Parkinson's with progressive supranuclear palsy-like symptoms. (130) St John's wort (*Hypericum perforatum*), useful for its amelioration of mild-to-moderate depression, was found to be associated with cataractogenesis. (131) Licorice (*Glycyrrhiza glabra*) has been reported to cause ocular migraine, transient visual loss, and central retinal vein occlusion. (132)

Coumarinic blood thinners

Garlic	Ginger	Ginkgo b.	Goldenseal	Echinacea	Passionflower
Chamomile	Parsley	Vanilla	Wild lettuce	Feverfew	Licorice
Flaxseed	Bilberr y	Papaya	Turmeric	Cayenne	Sage
Picorrhiza	Reichi	Turkeytail	Devils claw	Willow bark	Sunflower

Table 11. Herb-Drug Interactions

Ingestion and/or overdose can cause conjunctival, retinal and retrobulbar hemorrhages, hyphema, due to their inhibition of platelet aggregation. These herbs should not be taken along with conventional blood thinners and should be discontinued prior to any surgical procedure. (133) Plants, such as *Helianthus annuus*, whose fruit are sunflower seeds that contain high concentrations of vitamin E, can affect platelet aggregation and contribute to excessive bleeding when used with conventional blood thinners. (134)

Ephedra	Androstenedione	Aristolochic acids	Comfrey
Kava kava	Lipokinetix	Chaparral	Germander

Table 12. Botanicals or their ingredients banned or issued warnings by the FDA as hazardous or potentially dangerous

Ephedra (*Ephedra sinica*) used primarily in weight loss formulae, contains ephedrine, pseudoephedrine, and alkaloids, which can lead to high blood pressure, tachycardia, neuropathy, blurred vision, myopathy, tremors, memory loss, myocardial infarction, and death. (135) Androstenedione, found in pollen of the Scots pine (*Pinus sylvestris*) exhibits androgenic activity with side effects of blurred vision and temporary blindness. There are insufficient studies available to make definitive conclusions. Birthwort (*Aristolochia clematitis*) of the Aristolochia family, contains aristolochic acid which may have potent carcinogenic, hepatotoxic and nephrotoxic activity. Comfrey (*Symphytum officinale*) contains pyrrolizidine alkaloids, which are hepatotoxic when taken orally. Both may cause jaundiced eyes. (136) (137) Kava-kava (*Piper methysticum*) contains kavalactones, the active ingredient to treat social anxiety. It may cause visual impairment from mydriasis and reduced oculomotor balance. (138) Lipokinetix is another dietary weight loss agent, which contains usnic acid from the lichen, *Usnea barbata*. Along with chaparral (*Larrea tridentata*), it is known to be hepatotoxic and associated with jaundiced eyes. (139) (140) Germander (*Teucrium chamaedrys*) used primarily as a diet supplement, is highly toxic to the liver causing acute hepatitis, and should not be used in any form. (141)

Many food supplements have not been evaluated by the FDA. It is the responsibility of product manufacturer to ensure safety. Of those that have been evaluated and found ineffective or dangerous to health, the FDA has issued a warning which may range from mild, "This product is not intended to diagnose, treat, cure, or prevent any disease," to severe, "Not for human use" or "Illegal drug residue." For additional information, call:

US National Poison hotline 1-800-222-1222

References for Chapter Six:

1. Lisa Ganora 2008. Herbalchem Press, Louisville, Colorado. Herbal Constituents: Foundations of Phytochemistry:
2. "AERS Patient Outcomes by Year," Food and Drug Administraton (Washington, DC: U.S. Department of Health and Human Services, March 31, 2010.
3. Bronstein AC, et al, Clinical Toxicology (2009). 47, 911-1084. 2008 Annual Report of the American Association of Poison Control Centers' National Poison Data System (NPDS): 26th Annual Report.
4. Zafra-Stone S,et al. Mol Nutr Food Res. 2007 Jun; 51(6):675-83. Berry anthocyanins as novel antioxidants in human health and disease prevention.
5. Yao N, et al. J Agric Food Chem. 2010 Apr 28; 58(8):4731-6. Protective effects of bilberry (Vaccinium myrtillus L.) extract against endotoxin-induced uveitis in mice.
6. Song J, et al. Phytother Res. 2010 Apr; 24(4):520-4. Protective effect of bilberry (Vaccinium myrtillus L.) extracts on cultured human corneal limbal epithelial cells (HCLEC).
7. Matsunaga N, et al. Mol Nutr Food Res. 2009 Jul; 53(7):869-77. Bilberry and its main constituents have neuroprotective effects against retinal neuronal damage in vitro and in vivo.
8. Milbury PE, et al. Invest Ophthalmol Vis Sci. 2007 May; 48(5): 2343-9. Bilberry (Vaccinium myrtillus) anthocyanins modulate heme oxygenase-1 and glutathione S-transferase-pi expression in ARPE-19 cells.
9. Canter PH, Ernst E. Surv Ophthalmol. 2004 Jan-Feb; 49(1): 38-50. Anthocyanosides of Vaccinium myrtillus (bilberry) for night vision—a systematic review of placebo-controlled trials.

10. Zadok D, Leviy Y, Glovinsky Y. Eye (Lond). 1999 Dec;13 (Pt6): 734-6 The effect of anthocyanosides in a multiple oral dose on night vision.
11. Chung HK, et al. Arzneimittelforschung. 2005; 55(10): 573-80. Efficacy of troxerutin on streptozotocin-induced rat model in the early stages of diabetic retinopathy.
12. Deitre Z, et al. Clin Physiol Biochem. 1986; 4(2): 143-9. Studies on vascular permeability in hypertension: action of anthocyanosides.
13. Fursova AZh, et al. Adv Gerontol 2005; 16: 76-9. [Dietary supplementation with bilberry extract prevents macular degeneration and cataracts in senesce-accelerated OXYS rats].
14. Head KA. Altern Med Rev. 2001 Apr; 6(2): 141-66. Natural therapies for ocular disorders, part two: cataracts and glaucoma.
15. Rebecca L. Johnson & Steven Foster, Tierona Lowdog, MD, and David Keifer, MD. National Geographic Society 2010. National Geographic Guide to Medicinal Herbs.
16. Mix JA, Crews WD Jr. Hum Psychopharmacol. 2002 Aug; 17(6): 267-77. A double-blind, placebo-controlled, randomized trial of Ginkgo biloba extract EGb 761 in a sample of cognitively intact older adults: neuropsychological findings.
17. Ma K, et al. Acta Ophthalmol. 2010 Aug; 88(5) 553-7. The effect of ginkgo biloba on the rat ganglion cell survival in the optic nerve crush model.
18. Wimpissinger B, et al. Acta Ophthalmol Scand. 2007 Jun; 85(4):445-9. Influence of Ginkgo biloba on ocular blood flow.
19. Chung HS, et al. J Ocul Pharmacol Ther. 1999 Jun; 15(3): 233-40. Ginkgo biloba extract increases ocular blood flow velocity.
20. Jia LY, et al. Arch Ophthalmol. 2008 Dec; 126(12): 1700-6. Effect of topical Ginkgo biloba extract on steroid-induced changes in the trabecular meshwork and intraocular pressure.
21. Wu ZM, et al. Acta Pharmacol Sin. 2008 Sep; 29(9): 1042-50. Ginkgo biloba extract prevents against apoptosis induced by high glucose in human lens epithelial cells.
22. Quaranta L, et al. Ophthalmology. 2003 Feb; 110(2): 359-62. Effect of Ginkgo biloba extract on preexisting visual field damage in normal tension glaucoma.

23. Khoury R, et al. J Glaucoma. 2009 Sep; 18(7): 543-5. The association between self-reported glaucoma and ginkgo biloba use.
24. Jia Z, et al. Mol Vis. 2011 Jan 20; 17:210-7. Grape seed proanthocyanidin extract protects human lens epithelial cells from oxidative stress via reducing NF-kB and MAPK protein expression.
25. Barden CA, et al. Am J Vet Res. 2008 Jan; 69(1): 94-100. Effect of grap polyphenols on oxidative stress in canine lens epithelial cells.
26. Durukan AH, et al. J Cataract Refract Surg. 2006 Jun; 32(6): 1041-5. Ingestion of IH636 grape seed proanthocyanidin extract to prevent selenite-induced oxidative stress in experimental cataract.
27. Bagchi D, et al. Indian J Exp Biol. 2002 Jun; 40(6): 717-26. Mechanistic pathways of antioxidant cytoprotection by a novel IH636 grape seed proanthocyanidin extract.
28. Soares De Moura R, et al. J Pharmacol. 2002 Nov; 54(11): 1515-20. Antihypertensive, vasodilator and antioxidant effects of a vinifera grape skin extract.
29. Rohdewald P, Int J Clin Pharmacol Ther. 2002 Apr; 40(4):158-68. A review of the French maritime pine bark extract (Pycnogenol), a herbal medication with a diverse clinical pharmacology.
30. D'Andrea G. Fitoterapia. 2010 Oct; 81(7): 724-36. Pycnogenol: a blend of procyanidins with multifaceted therapeutic applications.
31. Steigerwalt R, et al. J Ocul Pharmacol Ther. 2009 Dec; 25(6): 537-40. Pycnogenol improves microcirculation, retinal edema, and visual acuity in early diabetic retinopathy.
32. Schönlau F, Rohdewald P. Int Ophthalmol. 2001; 24(3): 161=71. Pycnogenol for diabetic retinopathy. A review.
33. Sharma SC, Sharma S, Gulati OP. Phytother Res. 2003 Jan; 17(1): 66-9. Pycnogenol inhibits the release of histamine from mast cells.
34. Packer L, Rimbach G, Virgili F. Free Radic Biol Med. 1999 Sep; 27(5-6): 704-24. Antioxidant activity and biologic properties of a procyanidin-rich extract from pine (Pinus maritime) bark, pycnogenol.
35. Maccarone R, Di Marco S, Bisti S. Invest Ophthalmol Vis Sci. 2006 Mar; 49(3): 1254-61. Saffron supplement maintains morphology and function after exposure to damaging light in mammalian retina.

36. Yamauchi M, et al. Eur J Pharmacol. 2011 Jan 10; 650(1): 110-9. Crocetin prevents retinal degeneration induced by oxidative and endoplasmic reticulum stresses via inhibition of caspase activity.
37. Falsini B, et al. Invest Ophthalmol Vis Sci. 2010 Dec; 51(12): 6118-24. Influence of saffron supplementation on retinal flicker sensitivity in early age-related macular degeneration.
38. Cohen SY, et al. J Fr Ophthalmol. 2010 Apr; 33(4): 234-40. [Impact of eating habits on macular pathology assessed by macular pigment optical density measure].
39. Vibin M, et al. Curr Eye Res. 2010 Feb; 35(2): 99-107. Broccoli regulates protein alterations and cataractogenesis in selenite models.
40. Lans C, et al. J Ethnobiol Ethnomed. 2007 Feb 26; 3:11. Ethnoveterinary medicines used for ruminants in British Colombia, Canada.
41. Stoss M, et al. J Altern Complement Med. 2000 Dec; 6(6): 499-508. Prospective cohort trial of Euphrasia single-dose eye drops in conjunctivitis.
42. Preethi KC, Kuttan G, Kuttan R. Indian J Exp Biol. 2009 Feb; 47(2): 113-20. Anti-inflammatory activity of flower extract of Calendula officinalis Linn. And its possible mechanism of action.
43. Marinchev VN, et al. Oftalmol Zh. 1971; 26(3): 196-8. Use of Calendula for therapy of chronic inflammatory diseases of the eyelids and conjunctiva].
44. Corina P, et al. Oftalmologia. 1999; 46(1): 55-7. [Treatment with acyclovir combined with a new Romanian product from plants].
45. Chignell CF, et al. Photochem Photobiol. 2007 Jul-Aug; 83(4): 938-43. Photochemistry and phototoxicity of alkaloids from Goldenseal (Hydrastic Canadensis L.) 3: effect on human lens and retinal pigment epithelial cells.
46. Ormerod LD, et al. Am J Pathol. 1990 Nov; 137(5): 1243-52. Effects of altering the eicosanoid precursor pool on neovascularization and inflammation in the alkali-burned rabbit cornea.
47. Stozkowska W, Raczynska K. Przeol Lek. 2008; 65(5): 241-3. [Efficiency and application safety of Cepan cream. Observation of a new indication].

48. Geissberger P, Séquin U. Acta Trop. 1991 Feb; 48(4): 251-61. Constituents of Bidens pilosa L.: do the components found so far explain the use of this plant in traditional medicine?
49. Jäger AK, Hutchings A, van Staden J.J Ethnopharmacol. 1996 Jun; 52(2): 95-100. Screening of Zulu medicinal plants for prostaglandin-synthesis inhibitors.
50. Hamamelis in children with skin disorders and skin injuries: results of an observational study. Wolff HH, Keiser M. Eur J Pediatr. 2007 Sep; 166(9): 943-8.
51. Pain S, et al. Int J Cosmet Sci. 2011 Jun 29. doi: 10.1111/j.1468-2494. Surface rejuvenating effect of Achillea millefolium extract.
52. [No authors listed] Int J Toxicol. 2001; 20 Suppl 2: 79-84. Final report on the safety assessment of Yarrow (Achillea millefolium) Extract
53. Jin XH, et al. Exp Eye Res. 2006 May; 82(5): 860-7. Effects of blue honeysuckle (Lonicera caerula L.) extract on lipopolysaccharide-induced inflammation in vitro and in vivo.
54. Wojtowicz JC, et al. Cornea. 2011 Mar; 30(3): 308-14. Pilot, prospective, randomized, double-masked, placebo-controlled clinical trial of an omega-3 supplement for dry eye.
55. Pinheiro MN jr, et al. Arg Bras Oftalmol. 2007 Jul-Aug; 70(4): 649-55. [Oral flaxseed oil (Linum usitatissimum) in the treatment for dry-eye Sjögren's syndrome patients].
56. Barabino S, et al. Cornea. 2003 Mar; 22(2): 97-101. Systemic linoleic and gamma-linolenic acid therapy in dry eye syndrome with an inflammatory component.
57. Matsuda H, et al. Chem Pharm Bull (Tokyo). 2002 Jul; 50(7): 972-5. Medicinal flowers, VI. Absolute stereostructures of two new flavanone glycosides and a phenylbutanoid glycoside from the flowers of Chrysanthemum indicum L.: their inhibitory activities for rat lens aldose reductase.
58. Wei D, Li YH, Zhou WY. Zhongguo Zhong Xi Jie He Za Zhi. 2009 Jul; 29(7): 646-9. [Observation on therapeutic effect of runmushu oral liquid in treating xerophthalmia in post-menopausal women].

59. Kong FY, et al. J Ethnobiol Ethnomed. 2006 Jan 5; 2: 2. Parental use of the term "Hot Qi" to describe symptoms in their children in Hong Kong: a cross sectional survey "Hot Qi" in children.
60. Vlachojannis J, et al. Phytother Res. 2011 Jan 12. Doi: 10. 1002/ptr.3386. Willow species and Aspirin: Different Mechanism of Actions.
61. Aley, KO, et al. J Neuroscience 1998. Sep; 18(17): 7008-14. Nitric oxide signaling in pain and nociceptor sensitization in the rat.
62. Cady RK, et al. Headache. 2011 Jul; 51(7): 10788-86. A double-blind placebo-controlled pilot study of sublingual Feverfew and Ginger (LipiGesic™ M) in the treatment of migraine.
63. Agarwal KA, et al. Surg Endosc. 2011 Jun 14. Efficacy of turmeric (curcumin) in pain and postoperative fatigue after laparascopic cholecystectomy: a double-blind, randomized placebo-controlled study.
64. Hsu CH, Cheng AL. Adv Exp Med Biol. 2007; 595: 471-80. Clinical studies with curcumin.
65. Jiao Y, et al. Blood. 2009 Jan 8; 113(2): 462-9. Curcumin, a cancer chemopreventive and chemotherapeutic agent, is a biologically active iron chelator.
66. Singh S, et al. Phytomedicine. 2008 Jun; 15(6-7): 400-7. Boswellic acids: A leukotriene inhibitor also effective through topical application in inflammatory disorders.
67. Kar A, Menon MK. Life Sci. 1969 Oct 1; 8(19): 1023-8. Analgesic effect of the gum resin of Boswellia serrata.
68. Sengupta K, et al. Int J Med Sci. 2010 Nov 1; 7(6): 366-77. Comparative efficacy and tolerability of 5-Loxin and Aflapin against osteoarthritis of the knee: a double blind, randomized, placebo controlled clinical study.
69. Krishnaraju AV, et al. Toxicol Mech Methods. 2010 Nov' 20(9): 556-63.Safety and toxicological evaluation of Aflapin: a novel Boswellia-derived anti-inflammatory product.
70. Biju PG, et al. Mol Vis. 2007 Jul 12; 13: 1121-9. Drevogenin D prevents selenite-induced oxidative stress and calpain activation in cultured rat lens.

71. Anitha TS, et al. Biol Trace Elem Res. 2010 Oct 15. Prevention of selenite-induced cataractogenesis by an ethanolic extract of Cineraria maritime: an experimental evaluation of the traditional eye medication.
72. Gupta SK, et al. Curr Eye Res. 2005 Jul; 30(7): 583-91. Ocimum sanctum modulates selenite-induced cataractogenic changes and prevents rat lens opacification.
73. Gupta SK, et al. Biol Trace Elem Res. 2010 Sep; 136(3): 258-68. Trigonella foenum-graecum (Fenugreek) protects against selenite-induced oxidative stress in experimental cataractogenesis.
74. Gupta SK, et al. Ophthalmic Res. 2002 Jul-Aug; 34(4): 258-63. Green tea (Camillia sinensis) protects against selenite-induced oxidative stress in experimental cataractogenesis.
75. Yao K, et al. Mol Vis. 2008 Jan 31; 14: 217-23. Epigallocatechin gallate protects against oxidative stress-induced mitochondria-dependent apoptosis in human lens epithelial cells.
76. Manikandan R, et al. Fre Radic Biol Med. 2010 Feb 15; 48(4): 483-92. Curcumin prevents free radical-mediated cataractogenesis through modulations in lens calcium.
77. Manikandan R, et al. Curr Eye Res. 2010 Feb; 35(2): 122-9. Effect of curcumin on selenite-induced cataractogenesis in Wistar rat pups.
78. Saraswat M, et al. Mol Vis. 2010 Aug 10; 16: 1525-37. Antiglycating potential of Zingiber officinalis and delay of diabetic cataract in rats.
79. Rathi SS, et al. Phytother Res. 2002 Dec; 16(8): 774-7. Prevention of experimental diabetic cataract by Indian Ayurvedic plant extracts.
80. Srivastava Y, et al. Pharmacol Res Commun. 1988 Mar; 20(3): 201-9. Effect of Momordica charantia Linn. pomous aqueous extract on cataractogenesis in murrin alloxan diabetics.
81. Merritt, JC, Crawford WJ, Anduze AL, et al. American Academy of Ophthalmology presentation (Nov 1979) : 86:45. Effect of marijuana on intraocular and blood pressure in glaucoma.

82. Merritt JC, Crawford WJ, Anduze AL.Ophthalmology 1980 Mar:87(3):222-8. Effect of marijuana on intraocular and blood pressure in glaucoma.
83. Crawford WJ, Merritt JC. International J of Clinical Pharmacology and Biopharmacy 1979; 17:191-196. Effect of tetrahydrcannabinol on arterial and intraocular hypertension.
84. Merritt JC, et al. J Clin Pharmacol. 1981 Aug-Sep; 21 (8-9 Suppl): 4675-4715. Topical delta 9-tetrahydrocannabinol and aqueous dynamics in glaucoma.
85. Merritt JC, et al. Ophthalmic Research 1982; 14:124-128. Orthostatic hypotension after delta 9-THC marijuana inhalation.
86. Merritt JC, et al. Ann Ophthalmol 1980; 12:947-950. Oral delta 9- THC in heterogenous glaucomas.
87. Nadolska K, Gos R. Klin Oczna. 2008;110(10-12):392-6. [The role of endocannabinoid system in physiological and pathological processes in the eye].
88. Yazulla S. Prog Retin Eye Res. 2008 Sep; 27(5): 501-26. Endocannabinoids in the retina: from marijuana to neuroprotection.
89. Tirapelli CR, et al. Floterapia. 2010 Oct; 81(7): 690-702. Hypotensive action of naturally occurring diterpenes: a therapeutic promise for the treatment of hypertension.
90. Caprioli J, et al. Invest Ophthalmol Vis Sci. 1984 Mar; 25(3): 268-77. Forskolin lowers intraocular pressure by reducing aqueous inflow.
91. Pescosolido N, Librando A. Clin Ter. 2010; 161(3):e81-5. Oral administration of an association of forskolin, rutin and vitamins B1 and B2 potentiates the hypotonising effects of pharmacological treatments in POAG patients.
92. Head KA. Altern Med Rev. 2001 Apr; 6(2): 141-66. Natural therapies for ocular disorders, part two: cataracts and glaucoma.
93. Zhu MD, Cai FY. Zhonghua Yan Ke Za Zhi. 1991 May; 27(3): 174-8. The effect of Inj. Salviae Miltiorrhizae Co. on the retrograde axoplasmic transport in the optic nerve of rabbits with chronic IOP elevation].

94. Zhu MD, Cai FY. Chin Med J (Engl). 1993 Dec; 106(12): 922-7. Evidence of compromised circulation in the pathogenesis of optic nerve damage in chronic glaucomatous rabbit.
95. Agarwal R, et al. Ophthalmic Res. 2009; 42(2): 112-6. Intraocular pressure-lowering activity of topical application of Aegle marmelos fruit extract in experimental animal models.
96. Manjeshwar, SB, et al. Food Research International. 2011 Aug; 44(7);1768-75. Phytochemistry and medicinal uses of the bael fruit (Aegle marmelos Correa): a concise review.
97. Liu XP, et al. Zhong Yao Cai. 2009 May; 32(5): 736-40. Comparison of the antioxidant activity amongst Ginkgo biloba extract and its main components.
98. Chung HS, et al. J Ocul Pharmacol Ther. 1999 Jun; 15(3): 233-40. Ginkgo biloba extract increases ocular blood flow velocity.
99. Quaranta L, et al. Ophthalmology. 2003 Feb; 110(2): 359-82. Effect of ginkgo biloba extract on preexisting visual field damage in normal tension glaucoma.
100. Russo V, et al. Eur J Ophthalmol. 2009 May-Jun; 19(3): 331-6. Clinical efficacy of a ginkgo biloba extract in the treatment of allergic conjunctivitis.
101. Granger AS. Age Ageing. 2001 Nov; 30(6): 523-5. Ginkgo biloba precipitating epileptic seizures.
102. Leatherdale BA, et al. Br Med J (Clin Res Ed.) 1981. Jun 6; 282(6279): 1823-4. Improvement in glucose tolerance due to momordica charantia (Karela).
103. Ojewole JA, et al. Cardiovasc J S Afr. 2006 Sep-Oct; 17(5): 227-32. Hypoglycaemic and hypotensive effects of Momordica charantia Linn (Cucurbitaceae) whole-plant aqueous extract in rats.
104. Dans AM, et al. J Clin Epidemiol. 2007 Jun; 60(6): 554-9. The effect of Momordica charantia capsule preparation on glycemic control in type 2 diabetes mellitus needs further studies.
105. Ooi CP, Yassin Z, Hamid TA. Cochrane Database Syst Rev. 2010 Feb 17;(2): CD007845. Momordica charantia for type 2 diabetes mellitus.
106. Rathi SS, et al. Phytother Res. 2002 May; 16(3): 236-43. The effect of Momordica charantia and Mucuna pruriens in experimental

diabetes and their effect on key metabolic enzymes involved in carbohydrate metabolism.

107. Basch E, Gabardi S, Ulbricht C. Am J Health Syst Pharm. 2003 Feb 15; 60(4): 356-9. Bitter melon (momordica charantia): a review of efficacy and safety.
108. Shihabudeen MS, et al. Nutr Metab (Lond). 2011 Jun 29; 8(1): 46. Cinnamon extract inhibits alpha-glucosidase activity and dampens postprandial glucose excursion in diabetic rats.
109. Pham AQ, et al. Pharmacotherapy. 2007 Apr; 27(4): 595-9. Cinnamon supplementation in patients with type 2 diabetes mellitus
110. Kleefstra N, et al. Ned Tijdschr Geneeskd. 2007 Dec 22; 151(51): 2833-7. [Cinnamon: not suitable for treatment of diabetes mellitus].
111. Patil R, et al. Asian Pac J Trop Med. 2011 Apr; 4(4): 278-82. Isolation and characterization of anti-diabetic component (bioactivity-guided fractionation) from Ocimum sanctum L. (Lamiaceae) aerial part.
112. Misra H, et al. J Pharm Bioallied Sci. 2011 Apr; 3(2): 242-8. Antidiabetic activity of medium-polar extract from leaves of Stevia rebaudiana Bert. (Bertoni) on alloxan-induced diabetic rats.
113. Lailerd N, et al. Metab Clin Exp. 53(1): 101-7. Effects of stevoside on glucose transport activity in insulin-sensitive and insulin-resistant rat skeletal muscle.
114. Al-Romaiyan A, et al. Phytother Res. 2010 Sep; 24(9): 1370-6. A novel Gymnema sylvestre extract stimulates insulin secretion from human islets in vivo and in vitro.
115. Kar A, et al. J Ethnopharmacol. 2003 Jan; 84(1): 105-8. Comparative evaluation of hypoglycemic activity of some Indian medicinal plants in alloxan diabetic rats.
116. Shiyovich A, et al. Am J Med Sci. 2010 Dec; 340(6): 514-7. Toxic hepatitis induced by Gymnema sylvestre, a natural remedy for type 2 diabetes mellitus.
117. Rajasekaran S, et al. Pharmacol Rep. 2005 Jan-Feb; 57(1): 90-6. Antioxidant effect of Aloe vera gel extract in streptozotocin-induced diabetes in rats.

118. Botes L, et al. Molecules. 2008 Sep 12; 13(9): 2169-80. Phytochemical contents and antioxidant capacities of two aloe greatheadii var. davyana extracts.
119. Dey L, et al. Phytomedicine. 2003; 10(6-7): 600-5. Anti-hyperglycemic effects of ginseng: comparison between root and berry.
120. Lee WK, et al. Horm Metab Res. 2007 May; 39(5): 347-54. Ginsenoside Rh2 is one of the active principles of Panax ginseng root to improve insulin sensitivity in fructose-rich chow-fed rats.
121. Reeds DN, et al. Diabetes Care. 2011 May; 34(5): 1071-6. Ginseng and ginsenoside Re do not improve Beta-cell function or insulin sensitivity in overweight and obese subjects with impaired glucose tolerance or diabetes.
122. Udayakumar R, et al. Plant Foods Hum Nutr. 2010 Jun; 65(2): 91-8. Antioxidant effect of dietary supplement Withania somnifera L. reduce blood glucose levels in alloxan-induced diabetic rats.
123. Padiya R, et al. Nutr Metab (Lond). 2011 Jul 27: 8(1): 53. Garlic improves insulin sensitivity and associated metabolic syndromes in fructose fed rats.
124. Wu LY, et al. Eur J Nutr. 2004 Apr; 43(2): 116-24. Green tea supplementation ameliorates insulin resistance and increases glucose transporter IV content in a fructose-fed rat model.
125. Nayak BS, et al. Evid based Complement Alternat Med. 2011; 2011:875293. Hypoglycemic and hepatoprotective activity of fermented fruit juice of Morinda citrifolia (Noni) in diabetic rats.
126. Ziai SA, et al. J Ethnopharmacol. 2005 Nov 14; 102(2): 202-7. Psyllium decreased serum glucose and glycosylated hemoglobin significantly in diabetic outpatients.
127. Whiting DA, Bristow JH. S Afr Med J. 1975 Aug 16; 49(35): 1445-8. Dermatitis and keratoconjunctivitis caused by a prickly pear (Opuntia microdasys).
128. Raikhlin-Eisenkraft B, Bentur Y. J Toxicol Clin Toxicol. 2000; 38(3): 305-8. Ecbalium elaterium (squirting cucumber)—remedy or poison?

129. Fraunfelder FW. Am J Ophthalmol. 2004 Oct; 138(4): 639-47. Ocular side effects from herbal medicines and nutritional supplements.
130. Lannuzel A, et al. Brain 2007 Mar; 130(Pt 3); 816-27. Atypical parkinsonism in Guadeloupe: a common risk factor for two closely related phenotypes?
131. Booth JN 3rd, McGwin G. Curr Eye Res. 2009 Oct; 34(10): 863-6. The association between self-reported cataracts and St John's Wort.
132. Nencini C, et al. Eur Rev Med Pharmacol Sci. 2008 Sep-Oct; 12(5): 293-8. Retinopathy induced by drugs and herbal medicines.
133. Argento A, et al. Ann Ital Med Int. 2000 Apr-Jun; 15(2): 139-43. [Oral anticoagulants and medicinal plants. An emerging interaction].
134. Phang M, et al. Semin Thromb Hemost. 2011 Apr; 37(3): 199-208. Diet and thrombosis risk: nutrients for prevention of thrombotic disease.
135. Corrigan FM, Jennett J. Acta Psychiatr Scand. 2004 Aug; 110(2): 158. Ephedra alkaloids and brief relapse in EMDR-treated obsessive compulsive disorder.
136. Chen XW, et al. Chem Biol Interact. 2011 Jul 15; 192(3): 161-76. Herbal bioactivation, molecular targets and the toxicity relevance.
137. Mei N, et al. J Toxicol Environ Health B Crit Rev. 2010 Oct; 13(7-8): 509-26 Metabolism, genotoxicity, and carcinogenicity of Comfrey.
138. Garner LF, Klinger JD. J Ethnopharmacol. 1985 Jul; 13(3): 307-11. Some visual effects caused by the beverage kava.
139. Guo L, et al. J Environ Sci Health C Environ Carcinog Ecotoxicol Rev. 2008 Oct-Dec; 26(4): 317-38. Review of usnic acid and Usnea barbata toxicity.
140. Heron S, Yarnell E. J Altern Complement Med. 2001 Apr; 7(2): 175-85. The safety of low-dose Larrea tridentate (DC) Coville (creosote bush or chaparral): a retrospective clinical study.
141. Peréz Alvarez J, et al. Gastroenterol Hepatol. 2001 May; 24(5): 240-3. [Acute hepatitis due to ingestion of Teucrium chamaedrys infusion].

Exercise and Eye Health

Case Scenario One: "I am 52 years old and have just been diagnosed with early type 2 diabetes. I don't wish to take medications so my doctor agreed to let me try to control it with diet and exercise. I also have a family history of glaucoma. My last eye pressures were 22 and 23 mmHg but my visual fields and optic nerves were normal. I spend all day in front of a computer and am too tired in the evening to do much of anything. I know that I have to do something, but how exactly can exercise possibly help my eyes?"

Consequences of Not Exercising

Continuous daily physical activity is a major factor in most longevity studies. Direct biophysiological effects as well as indirectly contributing to good sleep and consequent cellular repair are two of the reasons given for the benefits of exercise in the elderly. (1) (2) Progressive body decline and loss of physiologic reserve in organs and systems accompanying natural ageing, are accelerated with immobility and lack of muscle activity. (3) Poor circulation especially in small peripheral vessels, which accompanies lack of exercise, can seriously affect the eyes and vision. Consequences of insufficient blood flow range from dark circles under and around the eyes due to pooling of venous blood and lymphatic stasis to retinal vessel sclerosis and occlusion, central serous chorioretinopathy, optic nerve atrophy, and ischemic optic neuritis. (4)

Improves ocular blood flow	Lowers eye pressure	Blood glucose control	Lowers blood pressure
Anti inflammation	Stress control	Muscle strength	Eliminates toxins

Table 1: Exercise Benefits for the Eyes:

How does exercise benefit the eyes?

Visual performance is impaired when ocular blood flow decreases. In a bicycling test, exercise increased ocular blood flow in the retinal and choroidal vessels, but not in the retinal arterioles and remained relatively stable during increased intensity. This was thought to be due to the autoregulatory mechanisms of the sympathetic nervous system. (5) Dynamic exercise (two-step test) increased blood flow in the retina in the immediate postexercise period and demonstrated a more persistent increase in choroid-retina, which again indicated a difference in the control mechanism of blood flow in the retina. (6) Nitric oxide is involved in the control of basal blood flow in the choroid, optic nerve, and retina through its vasodilator responses. During exercise, blood vessels use nitric oxide to signal the surrounding smooth muscles to relax, dilate, and increase blood flow. (7)

Another biochemical, endothelin-1, plays a role in choroidal blood flow by increasing the ocular perfusion pressure during isometric exercise. (8) After an initial increase in blood pressure leading to concomitant increases in ocular blood flow, autoregulation compensates to maintain a stable retinal blood flow. A normal retinal hemodynamic response to increases in perfusion pressure includes vasoconstriction, which normalizes blood flow. (9) Impairment of any of these pathways may be closely related to ocular diseases like glaucoma, diabetic retinopathy, and retinopathy of prematurity in which optic nerve and retinal ischemia are prominent.

Dynamic exercise results in an acute pronounced decrease in intraocular pressure (IOP) values of short duration, which return to pre-trained levels within a month. In primary open-angle glaucoma (POAG) patients, there was a stronger increase in choroidal blood flow in response to exercise than in controls, which indicated a possible impaired regulatory capacity. (10) (11) Short term but significant decreases in IOP, ocular pulse amplitude, and axial length were also found as results of exercise. (12) Further studies in exercise are needed to see if these physiologic and biochemical mechanisms can be of clinical benefit to glaucoma patients in longer term IOP control and even visual field protection and restoration.

Exercise reduces risk of cardiovascular disease, diabetes, hypertension, autoimmune, and neurodegenerative diseases, and indirectly reduces incidence of eye diseases.

Structured aerobic exercise and resistance training was associated with HbA1c reduction in patients with type 2 diabetes. The effect was greater when accompanied with dietary advice. (13) Exercise has beneficial effects on whole-body metabolism leading to enhanced insulin sensitivity, lowered glucose levels, and demonstrated prevention of diabetes. (14) (15)Physical activity, consisting of regular walking, lowered triglycerides, increased HDL, and was associated with significantly lowered risk of adverse cardiovascular events. (16) (17)

Low blood pressure and subsequent low ocular perfusion pressure have been associated with glaucomatous damage to the optic nerve head in a manner not completely understood. Increasing blood pressure has other deleterious effects and is not a viable solution. Maintaining optic nerve perfusion and IOP control remain the cornerstones of prevention of glaucoma progression. (18)

A healthy immune system is essential to prevention and improvement of eye diseases.

Regular moderate exercise exerts anti-inflammatory effects through modulation of immune mediators like, adipokines, cytokines, myokines, interleukin, and T and B cell functions, and increase in production of endocrine hormones.

Caution: Intense exercise can be detrimental in suppressing antibody production and inducing damaging stress factors, which may result in increased susceptibility to acute infections. Whether exercise is beneficial or detrimental depends on the intensity and the individual response. (19) (20)

Physical and emotional stresses lead to the release of numerous hormones, including cortisol, primarily from the adrenal glands. Prolonged elevated cortisol may induce oxidative damage to cellular constituents DNA and RNA and ultimately tissues and organs. Exercise releases endorphins, endogenous opioid peptides, from the pituitary gland and hypothalamus, which function to produce analgesia by redirecting pain-signaling molecules in the brain's neurons. By modulating and inhibiting cortisol activity, a protective effect and a feeling of well being is achieved. (21) (22) Exercise also leads to increases in connections between brain neurons, resulting in increased flow of oxygen-rich blood, which benefits the eyes. Changes in plasma glutathione and lipid peroxides are also evident in maintaining protective antioxidant activity. (23) a.m. affects an average of 30 percent of people in their nineties. People with an active lifestyle, defined as regular physical activity three times a week, leading up to this venerable age, showed a protective effect for incident exudative age-related macular degeneration, independent of other confounders. (24) Macular damage may be affected by the accumulation of waste products in the retina. Exercise accelerates the elimination of toxins.

How much exercise do we need?

Case Scenario Two: "Doctor A tells me I have to exercise. But I can't. This knee hurts, my heel hurts, I don't have time, (I really don't want to walk). Dr. X says I shouldn't bend down or do anything strenuous".

Unfortunately, laziness and perceived injury get confused with actual injury and lack of energy. Motivational treatment should be applied.

A recommended exercise regimen should be devised and structured according to needs of the individual, ability to perform, and mindset for fitness achievement. Telling a patient to exercise may not be enough. Showing, explaining, and providing a *prescription for exercise* will illuminate the facts on how, when, and why it works.

Morning exercise burns fat and is directed toward weight loss. Afternoon and evening exercise burn calories and carbohydrates most of which were acquired during the day. The most practical physical activity is walking.

Rx: Walk three to five miles for three to five times a week. Try to break a sweat and lengthen the time and distance as needed and as able.

Rx: Bike ten miles three to five times a week.

Rx: Swim one mile three to five times a week. Any and all variations can be implemented according to reasonable fitness criteria. The most important factor is *motivation* versus laziness. For those who cannot and will not get out and exercise, a complete regimen of *home exercises* to do while sitting on the couch can be provided.

Light	Slow dance	Low house chores	Gardening indoor
Moderate	Walking	Biking transport	Stretching/calisthenics
Tai chi/ Yoga	Gardening outdoor	High house chores	Jogging (+3mph)
Golf walking	Aquatic exercises	Gym/fitness ball	Home exercises
Vigorous	Running (+5mph)	Biking/cycling	Rowing
Swimming	Fast dance	Weight training	Most ball sports

Table 1: Types of Exercises for Continued Good Health:

Low household chores may consist of dusting, ironing, putting away groceries, taking out trash, washing dishes, and trimming plants. High chores are vacuuming, washing the car, washing windows, painting, and pushing a power mower.

Results:

Exercise produces cellular breakdown, which releases free radicals leading to mobilization of DNA components associated with antioxidant activity to engage in cell repair.Regular exercise builds resistance to oxidative stress and increases cellular capacity for self-protection and continuous repair.

Alternate activity with periods of recovery

Adverse Ocular Effects of Exercise:

Acute visual loss consisting of impairment in central visual acuity and reduced foveal sensitivity was associated with exercise in young patients with advanced glaucoma. Such patients should be advised to limit activities, which may bring on symptoms and adopt therapeutic measures to maintain ocular blood flow. (25)

Physicians should be aware that eye pressures may increase in association with additional pigment dispersion in pigmentary glaucoma if the pigment granules become dislodged and deposit on the trabecular meshwork and/or the iris contour is pushed forward during intense exercise particularly with head-down positions such as in yoga and stretching and jogging. Rather than avoiding exercise, pilocarpine therapy should be used to relieve the situation. (26) (27) Isometric exercises and weight lifting decrease intraocular pressure in normotensive and glaucomatous eyes. (28) IOP is elevated during Valsalva maneuver and maximum isometric contractions during heavy weight lifting presumably due to hypoxia/ischemia from breath holding. (29)

Aerobic exercise, reading, and both combined do not pose any risk for adverse events in normotensive and glaucoma patients. (30) (31)

Exercising in situations of extreme heat or cold is associated with significant changes in function of the immune system. Since other extraneous stress factors are present, the exact suppression mechanism and degree of effects are difficult to quantify. (32)

The physically fit patient is less likely to participate in risk-taking behavior, such as smoking and excessive alcohol intake, which can damage health. (33)

Eye Exercises and Ocular Muscle Strength:

The eye-hand coordination of elderly people who practiced *T'ai chi ch'uan* was better than that in controls. (34) Though both tai chi and swimming improve eye-hand coordination, TCC yielded better effects on dynamic balance than swimming. (35)

Though considered experimental, investigational, and largely unproven, orthoptic exercises were found to be an effective means of reducing symptoms in patients with exophoria from convergence insufficiency. The proximal and fusional components of the convergence muscles appear to be improved. (36)

References for Chapter Seven:

1. Panagiotakos DB, et al. Cardiol Res Pract. 2011 Feb 24; 2011:679187. Sociodemographic and lifestyle statistics of oldest old people (>80 years) living in Ikaria island: the Ikaria study.
2. Arakawa M, et al. Psychiatry Clin Neurosci. 2002 Jun; 56(3): 245-6. Comparative study on sleep health and lifestyle of the elderly in the urban areas and suburbs of Okinawa.
3. Ho AJ, et al. Hum Brain Mapp. 2011 Sep; 32(9): 1371-82. The effects of physical activity, education, and body mass index on the aging brain.
4. Beutelspacher SC, et al. Acta Ophthalmol. 2011 Mar 23; doi. 10 1111/j.1755-3768. Central serous chorioretinopathy shows reduced retinal flow circulation in retinal function imaging (RFI).
5. Hayashi N, Ikemura T, Soeya N. Eur J Appl Physiol. 2011 Mar 5. Effects of dynamic exercise and its intensity on ocular blood flow in humans.
6. Okuno T, et al. Eye (Lond). 2006 Jul; 20(7): 796-800. Ocular blood flow changes after dynamic exercise in humans.

7. Schmetterer L, Polak K. Prog Retin Eye Res. 2001 Nov; 20(6): 823-47. Role of nitric oxide in the control of ocular blood flow.
8. Fuchsjäger-Mayri G, et al. Invest Ophthalmol Vis Sci. 2003 Feb; 44(2): 728-33. Role of endothelin-1 in choroidal blood flow regulation during isometric exercise in healthy humans.
9. Harris A, et al. Graefes Arch Clin Exp Ophthalmol. 1996 Jul; 234(7): 440-4. Retinal blood flow during dynamic exercise.
10. Risner D, et al. J Glaucoma 2009 Aug; 18(6): 429-36. Effects of exercise on intraocular pressure and ocular blood flow: a review.
11. Portmann N, et al. Invest Ophthalmol Vis Sci. 2011 Aug 9. Choroidal blood flow response to isometric exercise in glaucoma patients and patients with ocular hypertension.
12. Read SA, Collins MJ. Eye (Lond). 2011 Jun; 25(6): 767-74. The short-term influence of exercise on axial length and intraocular pressure.
13. Umpierre D, et al. JAMA. 2011 May 4; 305(17): 1790-9. Physical activity advice only or structured exercise training and association with HbA1c levels in type 2 diabetes: a systemic review and meta-analysis.
14. O'Gorman DJ, Krook A. Med Clin North Am. 2011 Sep; 95(5): 953-69. Exercise and the treatment of diabetes and obesity.
15. Hu FB, et al. JAMA. 1999 Oct 20; 282(15): 1433-9. Walking compared with vigorous physical activity and risk of type 2 diabetes in women: a prospective study.
16. Hu FB, et al. Ann Intern Med. 2001 Jan 16; 134(2): 96-105. Physical activity and risk for cardiovascular events in diabetic women.
17. Durstine JL, et al. Sports Med. 2001; 31(15): 1033-62. Blood lipid and lipoprotein adaptations to exercise: a quantitative analysis.
18. Caprioli J, Coleman AL. Am J Ophthalmol. 2010 May; 149(5): 704-12. Blood pressure, perfusion pressure, and glaucoma.
19. Gleeson M, et al. Nat Rev Immunol. 2011 Aug 5. Doi: 10. 1038. The anti-inflammatory effects of exercise: mechanisms and implications for the prevention and treatmentof disease.
20. Walsh NP, et al. Exerc Immunol Rev. 2011; 17: 6-63. Position statement. Part One: Immune function and exercise.

21. Joergensen A, et al. PLoS One. 2011; 6(6): e20795. Association between urinary excretion of cortisol and markers of oxidatively damaged DNA and RNA in humans.
22. Harber VJ, Sutton JR. Sports Med. 1984 Mar-Apr; 1(2): 154-71. Endorphins and exercise.
23. Kretzschmar M, Müller D. Sports Med. 1993 Mar; 15(3): 196-209. Aging, training and exercise. A review of effects on plasma glutathione and lipid peroxides.
24. Knudtson MD, Klein R, Klein BE. Br J Ophthalmol. 2006 Dec; 90(12): 1461-3. Physical activity and the 15-year cumulative incidence of age-related macular degeneration: the Beaver Dam Eye Study.
25. Shah P, et al. Eye (Lond). 2001 Oct; 15(Pt5): 616-20. Exercise-induced visual loss associated with advanced glaucoma in young adults.
26. Jensen PK,et al. Am J Ophthalmol. 1995 Jul; 1120(1): 110-2. Exercise and reversed papillary block in pigmentary glaucoma.
27. Haynes WL, Johnson AT, Alward WL. Ophthalmology. 1992 Jul; 99(7): 1096-103. Effects of jogging exercise on patients with the pigmentary dispersion syndrome and pigmentary glaucoma.
28. Chromiak JA, et al. J Strength Cond Res. 2003 Nov; 17 (4): 715-20. Resistance training exercises acutely reduce intraocular pressure in physically active men and women.
29. Vieira GM, et al. Arch Ophthalmol. 2006; 124: 1251-1254. Intraocular pressure variation during weight lifting.
30. Natsis K, et al. BMC Ophthalmol. 2009 Aug 13; 9-6. Aerobic exercise and intraocular pressure in normotensive and glaucoma patients.
31. Medicina AM, et al. Arg Bras Oftalmol. 2007 Jan-Feb; 70(1): 115-9. [Effects of reading, exercise and exercise combined with reading on intraocular pressure for patients sustaining primary glaucoma (open angle) or ocular hypertension, both clinically controlled with topic medication].

32. Walsh NP, Whitham M. Sports Med. 2006; 36(11): 941-76. Exercising in environmental extremes: a greater threat to immune function?
33. Ortlepp JR, et al. Eur J Cardiovasc Prev Rehabil. 2004 Jun; 11(3): 192-200.Relationship between physical fitness and lifestyle behavior in healthy young men.
34. Pei YC, et al. J Formos Med Assoc. 2008 Feb; 107(2): 103-10. Eye-hand coordination of elderly people who practice Tai Chi Chuan.
35. Wong AM, et al. Arch Gerontol Geriatr. 2010 Sep 24. Does different exercise have the same effect on health promotion for the elderly? Comparison of training-specific effect of Tai Chi and swimming on motor control.
36. Aziz S, et al. Strabismus. 2006 Dec; 14(4): 183-9. Are orthoptic exercises an effective treatment for convergence and fusion deficiencies?

Stress and the Eye

Case Scenario One: I work on the computer all day and most of the night. When I get a chance, I workout at the gym until I'm overtired. My married life is not going so well and my coworkers are jealous of me and cause me grief. How can stress possibly hurt my eyes?

Physical and emotional stress, from both internal and external sources, often result in pronounced biochemical and physiological changes, which have profound effects on the body's systems. The hypothalamic-pituitary-adrenal (HPA) axis and the sympathetic nervous system (SNS) are the main pathways of the stress response system. The excessive release of oxidants and stress hormones has both a direct and indirect effect on the eyes. Release of adipokines and cytokines, can lead to a continuous stimulation of the system. (1) Oxidative stress results in the production of reactive oxygen species, like peroxides and free radicals, and concomitant reduction in antioxidant defenses, like glutathione, which damage cells directly through the processes of apoptosis and necrosis and lead to a reduction in the immune system's ability to repair. With its direct links to hypoxia and ischemia, stress plays a role in neurodegenerative, inflammatory, and vascular diseases, like sickle-cell anemia, hypertension, and diabetic retinopathy, which directly affect the eyes. With acute reaction to stress, the classic sympathetic response, the recovery is quick and usually without side effects. Chronic stress such as excessive and prolonged exposure to bright light and ultraviolet radiation, toxins, eyestrain, sleep deprivation, high blood pressure, high blood sugar, and excessive lipids, will stimulate the system to release continuous cortisol, which when secreted in excess, is associated with obesity, type 2 diabetes, cardiovascular complications and immune diseases. (2)

Biochemical Reaction to Stress:

Hydrogen peroxide	Superoxide	Hydroxyl radical	Organic hydroperoxide	Peroxy radical
Nitric oxide	Peroxy nitrite	Growth hormone	Epinephrine	Norepinephrine
Cortisol	Hypochlorous acid	Alkoxy radical	Endorphins	Prohibitin

Table 1: Prooxidants and Stress Hormones

The response to stress is modulated by both the mind and the body. The SNS reacts by secreting catecholamines for which there is a concomitant immunosuppression reaction, growth inhibition, and enhanced catabolism. Besides the immediate effects on blood flow and neuronal transmission, when chronic, DNA damage occurs, resulting in a more pronounced disease process. (3)

Exposure to constant light resulted in signaling mechanisms involving the protein, prohibitin, being led to retinal degeneration at the molecular level in mice. (4) Oxidative stress damage to the crystalline lens (cataract formation) was related to the mechanism of superoxide and hydrogen peroxide degradation of tissue lipids. (5) Light-induced injury led to retinal degeneration associated with changes in gene expression of iron metabolism proteins (ferritin) in the photoreceptor layers. (6) Stress-activated protein kinases have been implicated in dry eye and ocular surface disease by inducing transcription of related genes, which alter the production of inflammatory cytokines, tumor necrosis factor, and matrix metalloproteinases. (7) Researchers found a positive correlation between prolonged screen time (TV, videogame, and computer) and decrease in magnitude of retinal arterioles in a group of school-aged children. (8)

Blurred Vision	Headaches	Eye Twitching	Dizziness	Double Vision
Tired/Sore Eyes	Dry Eyes	Watery Eyes	Burning	Itching
Reduced Concentration	Change In Color Perception	Frequent Glasses Change	Slow Refocusing (Near To Far)	Lid Heaviness

Table 2. Symptoms of Stress-Related Eyestrain

Reading or working on the computer for ten hours or more will lead to stress-related eyestrain.

Acute stress is short term and the body's ability to react favorably with counteractive mechanisms is usually sufficient enough to prevent serious damage. The release of natural killer cells in the bloodstream, as well as increased blood flow, blood pressure, heart rate, and stress hormones, work to regulate and repair the initial injury. Multiple episodes can result in long term cellular, tissue, and organ destruction as seen with chronic stress.

Chronic stress is associated with the effects of excessive cortisol in raising blood glucose levels, enhancing the brain's use of energy and subsequent depletion, and major alterations in the immune system's ability to repair cells and react to inflammatory insults. The resulting imbalance between pro- and anti-inflammatory cytokines acts to redirect energy and resources from routine metabolic activity (digestive, reproductive, growth, and cognitive processes) to critical actions in the body. Epinephrine release coupled with lactic acid accumulation and subsequent release of leukotriene B4, prostaglandins, histamines, bradykinins, and hydrotryptamine lead to disruption of the immune system. Natural killer cell production is actually suppressed and the body becomes more susceptible to disease. In cases of exposure to toxic stress, opioids and more cortisol are released, which lead to suppression of all T-cells and further increase in disease susceptibility. (9)

Case Scenario Two: A 40-year-old obese female presents with blurred vision and all the signs and symptoms of pseudotumor cerebri. She is a schoolteacher who is single and has no social life, horrible eating habits, and she admits to having no physical activity. She is very dissatisfied with her condition, but has no motivation to change.

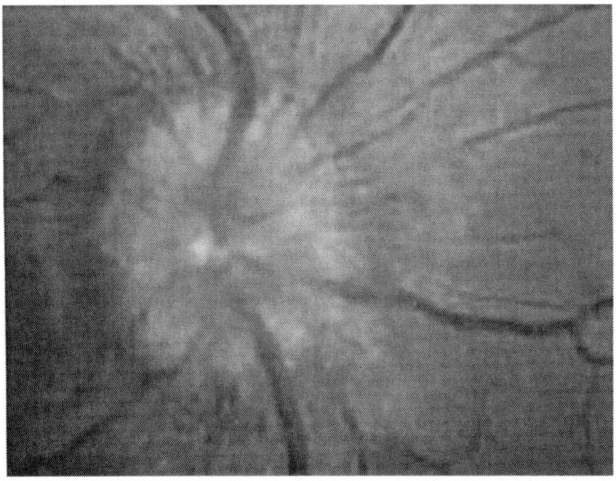

papilledema

Case Scenario Three: A 45-year-old male presents with light perception vision in the right eye and hand motion vision in the left eye of six months' duration due to bilateral cataracts. He was diagnosed with diabetes about two years prior, but had not taken his prescribed medications. He is overweight and lost his job when he could not function properly at the construction site.

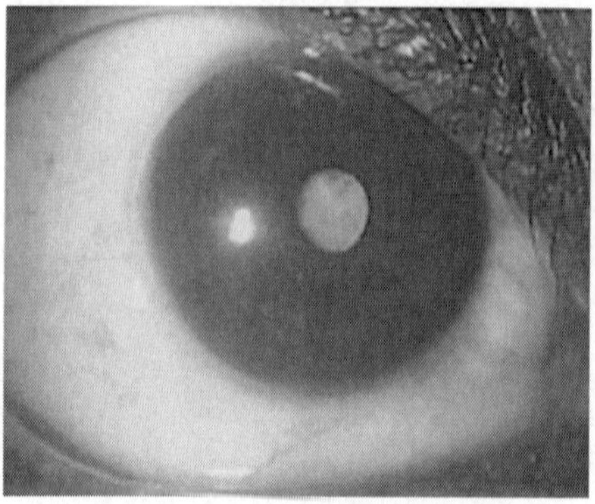

white hypermature cataract

Case Scenario Four: A 33-year-old male presents with blurred vision. He has recently relocated from the Midwestern United States to the Caribbean. He has a very fair skin complexion and admits to excessive sun exposure on the weekends and continuous computer work during the week. He is under extreme pressure to produce at his job as an engineer.

Central serous retinopathy (CSR), a condition in which there is a sensory detachment of the central retina, has been associated with type A personality in purpose-driven people under stress due to demanding occupations. It is associated with high levels of cortisol and corticosteroids in the bloodstream. Though most cases resolve without treatment, anti-inflammatory medications may be indicated for refractory cases. (10)

Emotional stress, categorized as the difference between feeling mad, angry, depressed, or disappointed versus happy, exuberant, optimistic, leads to hormonal releases, which may vary in different individuals and affect all the body systems. Some may release more cortisol and display anxiety and unease, while others may release hormones that lead to carbohydrate deficiency and subsequent craving. Positive and negative attitudes release differing amounts and varieties of stress hormones. Post traumatic stress disorder (PTSD) and its association with sleep deprivation through disruption of circadian rhythms, is dependent on a similar stress biochemistry. Oxidative damage at the cellular level is the common resulting pathology. (11)

Daytime emotional stress events can cause sleep disturbances. Though results may vary, there are disturbances in total sleep time, increased fragmentation, decreased sleep efficiency, and percentage of REM sleep, increased wake-after-sleep-onset latency and total time awake. These findings correlate well with negative emotions. (12) In addition, the IMPS (inventory to measure psychosocial stress) measured stress score was found to correlate positively with increased intraocular pressure in women, but not in men. This was apparently associated with the hypothalamic-pituitary-adrenal (HPA) axis and its hormonal reaction to stress. (13)

Case Scenario Five: An 80-year-old female with diminished vision due to long-term glaucomatous optic neuropathy presents with progressive visual field constriction. Being led into the examining room by her daughter, she complains of dimming vision and vocalizes only negative attributes of her condition. She complains of sleep deprivation and constant worry over the things she can no longer enjoy. Having had cataract/IOL and both laser and filtration surgeries done in both eyes successfully, her IOPs are 10 mmHg in each eye on brimonidine only. The next patient on the schedule, an 80-year-old male with a ten-year history of light perception vision in one eye and no light perception in the other, enters the examining room independently with his walking stick. He has bilateral optic atrophy and intraocular pressures of 13 and 11 mmHg, controlled with brimonidine drops twice daily. The patient sleeps well and awakens once only to relieve himself due to a mildly enlarged prostate gland. He enjoys his doctor's visit and talks about politics and friends. At his departure, he always states how he looks forward to the next visit.

Though not always significant on a man versus woman basis, these are examples of a difference in the pace of nerve degeneration, which may be associated with stress factors. Though the quantity of vision in both cases is poor, the quality of vision and function in patient two is far better.

Obstructive sleep apnea syndrome, associated with obesity with and without emotional stress, is implicated in retinal vein occlusion, glaucoma, papilledema, central serous retinopathy, and nonarteritic ischemic optic neuropathy. (14)

Patients with systemic diseases in which stress, anxiety and disability are prevalent, have reported *good* and *bad* vision days commensurate with physical and psychological levels of stress. In a group of patients with retinitis pigmentosa (RP), 87 percent to 93 percent of those who used therapies to alleviate stress, such as yoga, meditation, mind-body and energy therapies, acupuncture, and nutritional supplements, reported some visual improvement. (15) RP patients who kept their vision loss in perspective with a positive attitude, were better able to cope and manage the stress related to vision loss. (16)

Case Scenario Six: Two patients, a father and daughter, with retinitis pigmentosa are being followed for progression and complications. At 63 years old, he has given up on life, is on total disability, has a drug habit, and repeatedly uses terms like "I can't do this or that anymore." At 43 years old, she works as a secretary and repeatedly uses terms like "I will do this and that."

Bright Continuous Light	Ultraviolet Radiation	Hyperglycemia	Hyperlipidemia
Hypertension	Computer Eyestrain	Sleep Deprivation	Anxiety
Depression	Genetic Low Vision	Negative Attitude	Obesity

Table 3: Stressors and the Eye

Methods of Stress Control

The goal of organ and total body health is to keep stress hormone and oxidant levels under control. The body's reaction response to external and internal stressors must remain intact. The chronic stress response can be regulated by activating the relaxation response, the parasympathetic nervous system (PSNS).

The resulting reduction in cortisol release, increase in insulin production and reduction in oxygen species production will lead to a reduction in inflammation and disease susceptibility.

Basic strategies:	Balanced Diet	No Stimulants	Adequate Sleep	Positive Attitude
	Social Connections	Physical Activity	Resolve Conflicts	Be Realistic
CAM therapies:	Breathing Exercises	Guided Imagery	Biofeedback	Yoga
Eye exercises:	Palming	Near-Far Focus	Scanning	EMDR
Botanicals/Supplements:	Antioxidants	Adaptogens	Reduce Carbohydrates	B Vitamins
	Kava /Valerian	Omega-3 Fish Oil	CoenzymeQ10	Calcium/ Magnesium
Conventional therapies:	Tricyclic Antidepressants	Selective Serotonin Reuptakes	Anticonvulsants	Phenothiazines

Table 4: Stress Management Techniques:

Most of the above-listed therapies have been shown to improve immune function by increasing natural killer cell activity and the number of peripheral blood lymphocytes.

Though soothing and relaxing, there is no clinical evidence that meditation can change eye pressures in glaucoma. The clinical significance of the value of eye exercises is controversial as there are no clear evidence-based results from research trials at this time.

Computer Eyestrain Prevention**

1. Take a five-minute break every thirty minutes and rest eyes from VDT.
2. Position screen at eye level, twenty-two to twenty-six inches away (at arm's length to reduce electrical field to zero).
3. Face forward, keep neck relaxed.
4. Position keyboard so that elbows are bent ninety degrees and work without bending wrists.

5. Use a chair with back support, with feet resting on floor or footrest, and keep thighs parallel to floor.
6. If possible, step away from computer every hour for a fifteen-minute break.

**From the National Institute of Occupational Safety and Health Administration.

High levels of carbohydrates are associated with stressful situations. Maintaining these high levels with increased intake leads to a perpetuation of chronic stress and subsequent obesity, hyperglycemia, insulin resistance, hyperlipidemia, and immune system imbalance. (17)

Deep-breathing exercises relieve the sympathetic effects of stress by activating the parasympathetic system to reduce the release of proinflammatory oxygen free radicals and cortisol, to increase insulin and reduce hyperglycemia, and to restore homeostasis through a calming effect. The vagus (cranial nerve X) is the primary parasympathetic nerve, which when activated, slows the heart rate, dilates blood vessels, activates digestion, and stores energy. Abdominal breathing draws more blood to the lower lungs and more oxygen and nutrients to the tissues and organs. (18) (19) (20) Spontaneous sighing was found to be related to subjective relief of negative emotional states. (21)

Guided imagery has been found to provide significant stress-reduction benefits and is being used in many hospitals to help with preoperative and postoperative treatments. In a recent study, the RGI group showed less state anxiety, lower cortisol levels, and less surgical wound erythema than the control group. (22) Likewise, similar stress-reduction instructions given to pregnant women demonstrated significantly lower levels of stress, lower symptoms of depression and negative affect, and lower morning cortisol levels when compared to baseline. (23)

Biofeedback (autogenic therapy) exacting a system of relaxation exercises through the use of techniques of heart rate or thermal regulation was found to be helpful in reducing the effects of occupational stress and post-traumatic stress disorder. (24) (25)

In a group of thirty-five male volunteers, guided-imagery relaxation based on yoga exercises, reduced sympathetic activity as manifested by a reduction in heart rate, oxygen consumption, and increased breath volume, as seen when compared to baseline levels and controls. (26) Yoga reduced perceived stress and improved the autonomic response in a group of healthy pregnant women. (27) A group of visually impaired children showed significant decrease in their abnormal anxiety levels when they practiced yoga for three weeks, while a program of physical activity had much less effect. (28)

The palming exercise for eye relaxation involves rubbing the palms together to create heat and cupping them over the closed eyes for one to two minutes. Closing the eyes for two minutes in itself brings relaxation. The near-far focus exercises involve focusing on the thumb at close range then refocusing on an object at a distance. Convergence exercises and the breathing that accompanies this exercise are both physiologically and psychologically beneficial. Scanning the edges of objects in a room relaxes the eyes by keeping them moving in a loose and fluid way. Theoretically, this exercise is good despite the lack of clinical supporting evidence.

Eye movement desensitization and reprocessing (EMDR) is an integrative therapy that *unlocks* disturbing images or beliefs and reprocesses them. It was found to be of significant benefit in cases of post-traumatic stress disorder. (29)

A daily multivitamin with adequate amounts of ascorbic acid (vitamin C) included can help to minimize the damaging effects of oxidative stress on the body. (30) (31) Vitamin E in the form of tocotrienol, was shown to reduce the oxidative-nitrosative stress levels and inflammatory response; and improve neuropathic pain in diabetic rats at the molecular level, by inhibiting the reactive oxygen-nitrogen species, cytokines and apoptosis mechanism. (31) Vitamin B complex has been shown to have a calming effect on the sympathetic nervous system in cases of excessive work stress.

B vitamins have been found to be deficient in several cancer cases associated with oxidative stress (small cell lung cancer and liver cancer). (32) (33) (34)

In addition to the anti-inflammatory effects of omega-3 fish oils against oxidative stress on virtually all the layers of the eye, there is a protective effect at the RPE layer, which may be related to modifications in retinal prostaglandin metabolism. (35) (36)

The Cochrane Database of Systematic Review found that both Kava and valerian root extracts were effective in the symptomatic treatment of anxiety with relatively little side effects. (37) (38)

An earlier study found that both were useful in the treatment of stress and insomnia. (39)

A conflicting study found that both were no better than a placebo. (40)

A strict magnesium-calcium balance is required at the cellular level to regulate the stress-inflammation pathways (HPA and SNS). Magnesium deficiency activates oxidative stress to release excitatory proteins, which stimulate the immune system to produce the inflammation cascade, which in turn activates calcium to destabilize cellular metabolism. A magnesium-calcium balance is required to keep the stress-inflammation mechanism in check. (41) (42) Both optimal magnesium blood levels and low threshold calcium channels are needed for normal non-REM-to-REM-sleep regulation. (43) (44) Adequate magnesium-calcium sites are required for proper functioning of cardiac myofibrils, especially in the relaxation phase. Muscle relaxation during epidural anesthesia is significantly more effective when magnesium is added. (46) Oral magnesium supplementation appears to improve vascular function in elderly diabetic patients. (47) The careful regulation of the calcium-magnesium relationship is essential for the proper functioning of biochemical systems.

Adaptogens increase the body's resistance to physical, emotional, biological, and environmental stressors by regulating the hypothalamic-pituitary-adrenal (HPA) complex and adjusting imbalances in the immune system to prevent oxidative stress. The results are that they build stamina, ease anxiety, and enhance cognitive function.

Substantial scientific evidence exists for the therapeutic use of the ayurvedic herbal, ashwagandha (*Withania somnifera*) in reducing the reactive lipid peroxidation in stress-induced animals, as well as for normalizing physiological functions like insomnia and exhaustion for cases of chronic stress-related inflammation, immune system deficits, and neurodegenerative diseases. (48) (49)

Panax ginseng (Chinese) is known for its activity in the restoration of body vitality, immune system-boosting properties, positive effect on prevention of atherosclerosis through maintenance of endothelial cell function and improvement in cognitive function. Its main action is on the hypothalamic-pituitary-adrenal (HPA) system in the regulation of oxidative stress. *Panax quinquefolius* (American) prevented glucose-induced oxidative stress damage to umbilical vein endothelial cells by inhibiting the accumulation of reactive oxygen species, generation of superoxide anion and localized DNA damage through its antioxidant properties. (50) (51) (52)

There was a beneficial effect after administering Eleutheroside E, a component of *Eleutherococcus senticosus*, also known as Siberian ginseng, to sleep-deprived mice by its activity on restoring monoamines in the hypocampus. Its effects on chronic fatigue, stress, and insomnia in elderly patients were more positive than those of placebo. (53) (54) (55)

Coenzyme Q10 (CoQ10) is a vital nutrient for cellular energy production taking place in the mitochondria via electron transfer across membranes. Metabolized in all body tissues, it is an antioxidant with a quinine chemical group and is best absorbed as a supplement when taken orally as ubiquinol. It is found in best quantities in meat, fish, parsley, broccoli, cauliflower, and avocado. CoQ10 has been found to protect the hypocampal neurons from neurotoxicity due to oxidative stress, lower both systolic and diastolic blood pressures, heal or reduce radiation damage, improve heart health in chronic heart failure, prolong lifespan in rats and nematodes, and reduce the progression of Parkinson's by 44 percent when taken at a dosage of 1200 mg per day. Its possible mechanism of action of prevention and repair of stress-induced injuries appeared to be through the modulation of LOX-1-mediated reactive oxygen species generation via specific signaling pathways. (56) (57)

Conventional antidepressants for stress control may be overprescribed and overused in our western society. The tricyclic antidepressants (TCA) are recommended for sleep deprivation, post-traumatic sleep disorders, and anxiety and have the potential to induce numerous ocular side effects, such as chronic uveitis and reduced accommodation. The antidepressant/anticonvulsant drug, topiramate, used for migraine headaches, resulted in angle-closure glaucoma, myopic shift, and an increase in retinal nerve fiber layer thickness. Allergic-type reactions in which the lens and ciliary body were displaced have also been reported. Long-term use and high doses of phenothiazines like chlorpromazine and thorazine, were strongly associated with lid and conjunctival discoloration, cataractogenesis, and retinopathy.

Other visual problems of note were eye movement disorders, decreased color perception, and reduced contrast sensitivity. (58) (59) (60) (61)

The selective serotonin reuptake inhibitors (SSRIs) such as fluoxetine can cause mydriasis, which may promote angle-closure glaucoma in susceptible individuals. (62)

The long-term use of anxiety-relieving benzodiazeprines showed mild changes in the ERG pattern and elicited complaints of blurred vision and difficulty reading, but had no pathological effect on the retina. (63)

Physicians and patients need to be aware of the strong systemic and ocular side effects of conventional drugs, as well as similar side effects from supplements. Though there may be a place for herbal remedies in the treatment of anxiety-related stress and insomnia, reliance on supplements for stress control is not good practice and is not recommended. The effects of acute and chronic stress on the eye and their direct association with dysfunction and disease should be taken into account in all cases of inflammation and immunity. Dietary adjustments, avoidance of stressful situations and basic coping appear to be the most efficient and safest approaches to stress control.

References for Chapter Eight:

1. Krou I, Tsigos C. Curr Opin Pharmacol. 2009 Dec; 9(6): 787-93. Stress hormones: physiological stress and regulation of metabolism.
2. British Journal of Haematology 132 (1): 108-113. Red blood cells, platelets and polymorphonuclear neutrophils of patients with sickle cell disease exhibit oxidative stress that can be ameliorated by antioxidants.
3. Hara MR, et al. Nature. 2011 Aug 21; 477(7364): 349-53. A stress response pathway regulates DNA damage through Beta2-adrenoreceptors and Beta-arrestin-1.
4. Lee H, et al. Int J Biol Macromol. 2010 Dec 1; 47(5): 685-90. Prohibitin as an oxidative stress biomarker in the eye.
5. Varma SD, et al. Curr Eye Res. 1984 Jan; 3(1): 35-57. Oxidative stress on lens and cataract formation: role of light and oxygen.
6. Picard E, et al. Invest Ophthalmol Vis Sci. 2011 Mar 10; 52(3): 1261-74. Light-induced retinal degeneration correlates with changes in iron metabolism gene expression, ferritin level, and aging.
7. Pfugfelder SC, et al. Ocul Surf. 2005 Oct; 3(4): 154-7. Stress-activated protein kinase signaling pathways in dry eye and ocular surface disease.

8. Gopinath B, et al. Arterioscler Thromb Vasc Biol. 2011 May; 31(5): 1233-9. Influence of physical activity and screen time on the retinal microvasculature in young children.
9. Cohen S, Tyrrell DA, Smith AP. N Engl J Med. 1991 Aug 29: 325(9): 606-12. Psychological stress and susceptibility to the common cold.
10. Wang M, et al. Acta Ophthalmol. 2008 Mar; 86(2): 126-45. Central serous chorioretinopathy.
11. Richards RS, Nwose EU, Bwititi P. Med Hypotheses. 2011 Oct; 77(4): 605-9. Biochemical basis of circadian rhythms and diseases: with emphasis on post-traumatic stress disorder.
12. Vandekerckhove M, et al. Psychophysiology. 2011 Sep 6; 1469-8986. The role of presleep negative emotion in sleep physiology.
13. Yamamoto K, et al. J Physiol Anthropol. 2008 Jan; 27(1): 43-50. The relationship between IMPS-measured stress score and intraocular pressure in public school workers.
14. Leroux les Jardins G, et al. J Fr Ophtalmol. 2009 Jun; 32(6): 420-4. [Retinal vein occlusion and obstructive sleep apnea syndrome].
15. Kiser AK, Dagnelie G. Clin Exp Optom. 2008 Mar; 91(2): 166-76. Reported effects of non-traqditional treatments and complementary and alternative medicine by retinitis pigmentosa patients.
16. Bittner AK, Edwards L, George M. Optometry. 2010 Sep; 81(9): 461-8. Coping strategies to manage stress related vision loss and fluctuations in retinitis pigmentosa.
17. Markus CR, Biol Psychol. 2007 Sep; 76(1-2): 83-90. Effects of carbohydrates on brain tryptophan availability and stress performance.
18. Virgerhoets AJ. Int J Psychosom. 1985; 32(3): 28-34. The role of the parasympathetic division of the autonomic nervous system in stress and the emotions.
19. Martarelli D, et al. J Altern Complement Med. 2011 Jul; 17(7): 623-8. Diaphragmatic breathing reduces postprandial oxidative stress.
20. Brown RP, Gerbarg PL, J Altern Complment Med. 2005 Aug; 11(4): 711-7. Sudarshan Kriya Yogic breathing in the treatment

of stress, anxiety, and depression. Part II-clinical applications and guidelines.

21. Vlemincx E, et al. Physiol Behav. 2010 Aug 4; 101(1): 67-73. Take a deep breath: the relief effect of spontaneous and instructed sighs.
22. Holden-Lund C. Res Nurs Health. 1088 Aug; 11(4): 235-44. Effects of relaxation with guided imagery on surgical stress and wound healing.
23. Urizar GG Jr, et al. Biol Psychol. 2004. Impact of stress reduction instructions on stress and cortisol levels during pregnancy.
24. Stein F. Work. 2001; 17(3): 235-245. Occupational stress, relaxation therapies, exercise and biofeedback.
25. Hickling EJ, et al. Biofeedback Self Regul. 1986 Jun; 11(2): 125-34. Treatment of posttraumatic stress disorder with relaxation and biofeedback training.
26. Vempati RP, Telles S. Psychol Rep. 2002 Apr; 90(2): 487-94. Yoga-based guided relaxation reduces sympathetic activity judged from baseline levels.
27. Satyapriya M, et al. Int J Gynaecol Obstet. 2009 Mar; 104(3): 218-22.Effect of integrated yoga on stress and heart rate variability in pregnant women.
28. Telles S, Naveen KV. Indian J Med Sci. 1997 Apr; 51(4):123-7. Yoga for rehabilitation: an overview.
29. Lee GK, Beaton RD, Ensign J. J Psychosoc Nurs Ment Health Serv. 2003 Jun; 41(6): 22-31. Eye movement desensitization and reprocessing. A brief and effective treatment for stress.
30. Kashino G, et al. Free Radic Biol Med. 2003 Aug 15; 35(4):438-43. Relief of oxidative stress by ascorbic acid delays cellular senescence of normal human and Werner syndrome fibroblast cells.
31. Kuhad A, Chopra K. Neuropharmacology. 2009 Sep; 57(4): 456-62. Tocotrienol attenuates oxidative-nitrosative stress and inflammatory cascade in experimental model of diabetic neuropathy.
32. Stough C, et al. Hum Psychopharmacol. 2011 Sep 8. 1229 The effect of 90 day administration of a high dose vitamin B-complex on work stress.

33. Tsao Sm, Yin MC, Liu WH. Nutr Cancer. 2007; 59(1):8-13. Oxidant stress and B vitamins status in patients with non-small lung cancer.
34. Lin CC, Yin MC. Eur J Nutr. 2007 Aug; 46(5): 293-9. B vitamins deficiency and decreased anti-oxidative state in patients with liver cancer.
35. Barbosa DS, et al. Nutrition. 2003 Oct; 19(10): 837-42. Decreased oxidative stress in patients with ulcerative colitis supplemented with fish oil omega-3 fatty acids.
36. Schnebelen C, et al. Nutr Res. 2011 Apr; 31(4):286-95. Dietary polyunsaturated fatty acids reduce retinal stress induced by an elevation of intraocular pressure in rats.
37. Pittler MH, Ernst E. Cochrance Database Syst Rev. 2003; (1): CD003383. Kava extract for treating anxiety.
38. Miyasaka LS, et al. Cochrane Database Syst Rev. 2006 Oct18; (4): CD004515. Valerian for anxiety disorders.
39. Wheatley D. Phytother Res. 2001 Sep; 15(6): 549-51. Kava and valerian in the treatment of stress-induced insomnia.
40. Jacobs BP, et al. Medicine (Baltimore). 2005 Jul; 84(4): 197-207. An internet-based randomized, placebo-controlled trial of kava and valerian for anxiety and insomnia.
41. Rayssiguier Y, et al. Magnes Res. 2010 Jun; 23(2): 73-80. Magnesium deficiency and metabolic syndrome: stress and inflammation may reflect calcium activation.
42. Peng TI, Jou MJ. Ann N Y Acad sci. 2010 Jul; 1201: 183-8. Oxidative stress caused by mitochondrial calcium overload.
43. Chollet D, et al. Behav Genet. 2001 Sep; 31(5): 413-25. Magnesium involvement in sleep: genetic and nutritional models.
44. Astori S, et al. Proc Natl Acad Sci USA. 2011 Aug 16; 108(33): 13823-8. The CaV3.3 calcium channel is the major sleep spindle pacemaker in thalamus.
45. Fuchs F, Grabarek Z. Biochem Biophys Res Commun. 2011 May 20; 408(4): 697-700. The Ca2+/Mg2+ sites of troponin C modulate crossbridge-mediated thin filament activation in cardiac myofibrils.

46. Yousef AA, Amr YM. Int J Obstet Anesth. 2010 Oct; 19(4): 401-4. The effect of adding magnesium sulphate to epidural bupivacaine and fentanyl in elective caesarean section using combined spinal-epidural anaesthesia: a prospective double blind randomized study.
47. Barbagallo M, et al. Magnes Res. 2010 Sep; 23(3): 131-7. Oral magnesium supplementation improves vascular function in elderly diabetic patients.
48. Dhuley JN. J Ethnopharmacol. 1998 Mar; 60(2): 173-8. Effect of ashwagandha on lipid peroxidation in stress-induced animals.
49. Ven Murthy MR, et al. Cent Nerv Syst Agents Med Chem. 2010 Sep 1; 10(3): 238-46. Scientific basis for the use of Indian ayurvedic medicinal plants in the treatment of neurodegenerative disorders; ashwagandha.
50. Zeng Y, Song JX, Shen XC. Phytother Res. 2011 Sep 16.1002/3587. Herbal Remedies Supply a Novel Prospect for the Treatment of Atherosclerosis: A Review of Current Mechanism Studies.
51. Liu L, et al. Zhongguo Zhong Yao ZA Zhi. 2011 May; 36(10): 1342-7. [Effects of ginsenosides on hypothalamic-pituitary-adrenal function and brain-derived neurotrophic factor in rats exposed to chronic unpredictable mild stress].
52. Sen S, et al. Phytomedicine. 2011 Aug 12. American ginseng (Panax quinquefolius) prevents glucose-induced oxidative stress and associated endothelial abnormalities.
53. Huang LZ, et al. Eur J Pharmacol. 2011 May 11; 658 (2-3): 150-5. The effect of Eleutheroside E on behavioral alterations in murine sleep deprivation stress model.
54. Hartz AJ, et al. Psychol Med. 2004 Jan; 34(1): 51-61. Randomized controlled trial of Siberian ginseng for chronic fatigue.
55. Cicero AF,et al. Arch Gerontol Geriatr Suppl. 2004; (9):69-73. Effects of Siberian ginseng (Eleutherococcus senticosus maxim.) on elderly quality of life: a randomized clinical trial.
56. Won R, Lee KH, Lee BH. Neuroreport. 2011 Oct 5; 22(14): 721-6. Coenzyme Q10 protects neurons against neurotoxicity in hippocampal slice culture.

57. Tsai KL, et al. Mol Nutr Food Res. 2011 Aug 3. Coenzyme Q10 suppresses oxLDL-induced endothelial oxidative injuries by the modulation of LOX-1-mediated ROS generation via the AMPK/PKC? NADPH oxidase signaling pathway.
58. Aurora RN, et al. J Clin Sleep Med. 2010 Aug 15; 6(4): 389-401. Best practice guide for the treatment of nightmare disorder in adults.
59. Richa S, Yazbek JC. CNS Drugs. 2010 Jun 1; 24(6): 501-26. Ocular adverse effects of common psychotropic agents: a review.
60. Ozturk BT, et al. Curr Eye Res. 2011 Jan; 36(1): 47-52. Ocular changes associated with topiramate.
61. Valentine M, Jardine P. Br Med J. 1966 Sep 3; 2(5513): 586. Phenothiazines and eye complications.
62. Costagliola C, et al. Curr Neuropharmacol. 2008 Dec; 6(4): 293-310. Selective serotonin reuptake inhibitors: a review of its effects on intraocular pressure.
63. Stafanous SN, et al. Doc Ophthalmol. 1999; 99(1): 55-68. The effect of long-term use of benzodiazeprines on the eye and retina.

Energy Medicine and the Eye

Case Scenario One: A 48-year-old female complains that her eyes always feel tired, painful, and have difficulty focusing after reading for a short time. Her glasses were recently updated and found to be satisfactory. She admits to not getting enough sleep, but does not wish to take sedatives or antidepressants. She asks "What else can I do? How can energy medicine help my eyes?"

All organisms rely on the generation of energy to sustain life. Energy is that special quality of life we philosophically refer to as vital force—a combination of mind, body, and soul by which organisms derive their consciousness. The principles of energy medicine originate in quantum physics, a discipline for which the body is perceived as an electromagnetic field existing in an electromagnetic environment. Conversely, no living force has conclusively been found at our level of scientific experimentation. However, we do have evidence-based studies showing that electrical and magnetic forces exert some activity on the physiology of the body.

Known forms of energy such as light, UV radiation, color, and electromagnetic therapy for which there is a demonstrated relationship to the functioning of the body are referred to as veritable therapies. Biofield energy healing falls under the heading of putative therapies and relates to the eye in its alleviation of pain.* The biofield hypothesis explains the interaction of objects or fields with the organism and resultant effects. (1) (2)

In randomized double-blind studies, various forms of distant healing, though not absolutely conclusive in regards to cause and effect, have shown significant improvement when compared to controls. In other studies, there were no improvements in selected outcomes. Studies were done with HIV patients and included both subjective and objective findings. (3) (4)

Pain Management

Low-level laser therapy during radiotherapy was found to be effective in controlling the intensity of pain in the treatment of mucositis. (5) Unfiltered or misapplied UV radiation is damaging to eyes and skin. (6)

Pain induced by nociceptive stimulation (CO2 laser) was relieved by concurrently adopted sensory stimuli from vibration and movement, and gave positive alleviation. Some Reiki studies showed a modest effect for pain relief when compared to placebo and other studies on touch therapies were inconclusive. (7) (8) There are no specific studies on energy medicine available for relief of eye pain.

**Theorized forms of energy not yet substantiated by scientific investigation are beyond the scope of this book and will not be addressed.*

Light Therapy

Skin disease	Sleep disorders	Seasonal affective disorders
Non-seasonal depression	Psychiatric disorders	Wound healing
Neonatal jaundice	Age-related macular degeneration	Parkinson's disease
Sinus-related disease	Hirsuitism	Immune diseases

Table 1. Disorders Amenable to Phototherapy

Certain living cells convert light into energy, which can be used to treat several disorders. Daylight, lasers, light-emitting diodes, fluorescent lamps, dichroic lamps, and bright, full-spectrum light are administered at specific times and for specified durations.

Vision is initiated by the stimulation of visual pigments through photoisomerization, which is driven by both thermal and photon energy. The reaction of pigments gives rise to the visual spectrum as well as infrared and ultraviolet light, radiation, and vibrational energy. (9)

Skin disorders like psoriasis, acne vulgaris, vitiligo, lichen planus, mycosis fungoides, and eczema respond well to light therapy using wavelengths of UV-A between 315 and 400 nm, and UV-B between 280 and 315 nm. Light is directed to the specific affected area. Light therapy for the regulation of circadian rhythm uses a light box, which emits up to 10,000 lux of energy, or a lower intensity of specific wavelengths. Selection depends on clinical efficacy, safety, and visual comfort. Fluorescent lamps that give off white light or blue light at 470 nm are used to manipulate levels of the sleep-regulating hormone, melatonin. Timing is important to regulate the sleep-wake phases and achieve the maximum effect. Direct sunlight, manipulated by a computer-controlled heliostat, can be used as light therapy in the treatment of seasonal affective disorders (SAD) in which both rods and cones are stimulated. (10) (11) This arrangement is effective when dealing with aberrant reactions ranging from allergies to shift work. The use of bright light, along with melatonin, timed exercise and selective diets, and social stimuli, affecting the suprachiasmatic nucleus of the hypothalamus, is currently under investigation for the treatment of jet lag. (12) (13)

Light-emitting diodes (LED) blue light, such as that emitted by some computers, was also found to suppress melatonin in its treatment of seasonal affective disorders. (14)

In relation to the physiological reaction to light, there is a connection between cones in the retina and the thalamus in producing behavior and the hypothalamus-pituitary-adrenal (HPA) system, in the stress response. Red light induces oxidative stress and elicits higher levels of melatonin release than the other spectra. (15)

Light therapy can be used in the treatment of non-seasonal depression, bipolar disorders, postpartum depression, and other major depressive disorders, with fairly successful results. Optimal dosing and treatment time of day must be individualized and is often accompanied b antidepressant medication. Caution: Side effects include possible hypomania and autonomic hyperactivation. (16) (17) (18) Though modern techniques of phototherapy are considered safe when properly administered, there is a higher risk of adverse effects when used with photosensitizing drugs.

LEDs in both the near-infrared and green wavelengths, appear to boost energy levels within cells resulting in accelerated fibroblast proliferation beneficial in wound healing. (19) (20) (21)

The use of low-level laser therapy (LLLT) for cutaneous wound healing has produced positive results especially in animal studies where there was reduced inflammation and faster progression through the healing phases, but FDA approval is not forthcoming due to lack of sufficient evidence in support of widespread use. More exact studies are needed that would pinpoint the biological processes involved in achieving these cellular effects. (22) (23)

Phototherapy is now the standard of treatment for infants with neonatal jaundice due to hyperbilirubinemia. The application of blue or white light (bili light) produces a prolonged reduction in bilirubin levels through isomerization into compounds more amenable to excretion in the urine and stool. (24) (25)

Bright light therapy has been shown to improve bradykinesia and rigidity and reduce agitation, dyskinesia and psychiatric side effects, but had no effect on the tremors of Parkinson's disease. Dosages of L-dopamine were able to be reduced when by the action of light therapy on suppressing melatonin secretion. (26) (27)

Uveitis	Vitreitis	Retinitis	Manic tendency
Photosensitive skin conditions	Photosensitive herbs(St John's wort)	Porphyria	Methotrexate & chloroquine

Table 2. Conditions Associated with Phototoxicity:

The mechanism of action of the application of light in reducing inflammation is through lowering levels of prostaglandins, cytokines, and circulating inflammatory cells by the transfer of energy from physical to chemical effect. It stimulates the mitochondria to release adenosine triphosphate to increase oxygen reactive species, which influences redox signaling, resulting in the proliferation of cells and changes in biochemical constituents of the affected cells. Likewise, overstimulation of these mechanisms can lead to symptoms of nervousness, anxiety, headache, and nausea.

Photodynamic therapy with verteporfin, in which the drug was administered intravascularly and activated with light, was shown to stabilize choroidal neovascularization in age-related macular degeneration, and gave rise to the more advanced ranibizumab use in giving better visual results. (28)

Exposure to ultraviolet radiation can have a two-fold effect depending on intensity and response; may cause photokeratitis, uveitis, pterygium, cataract, malignancies, and infections from immunity suppression, or it may lead to antigen-specific immune responses, which may benefit the very same detrimental conditions. (29) (30) (31)

The use of colored lenses (yellow and orange) by patients for age-related macular degeneration showed some improvement in contrast sensitivity. Gray lenses helped in the presence of glare, but red lenses decreased vision and peripheral sensitivity. The results were subjective, but warrant further study. (32)

Color Therapy and Glasses

There are seven visible colors in the optical spectrum and a range of invisible infrared and ultraviolet wavelengths to which body tissues are sensitive. The eye converts light into energy, which goes to the CNS and affects all systems at the cellular and hormonal levels. Color is discerned in the hypothalamus, pineal gland, and pituitary (stress response); all of which regulate hormone production. Color has a measurable effect on mood and emotions and influence conditions of insomnia, depression, and anxiety. Though conclusive evidence is still limited, specific environmental stimuli like bright red light for excitation and blue light for a calming effect, have been found to affect individual stress levels. (33) (34) (35) (36) Studies have shown that wearing lenses with medical filters in the range of green-yellow wavelengths (565–570 nm) was successful in slowing down the progression of age-related macular degeneration and a positive effect on their depression. Colors generate electrical impulses, which activate biochemical and hormonal processes. Warm colors increased respiratory movements, frequency of eye blinks, cortical activation, and palmar conductance, all stimulatory activities reactions of the autonomic nervous system. Cool colors acted as relaxants in anxious individuals, lowered blood pressure, apparently relieved tension and muscle spasms, and reduced eye-blinking frequency. The mode of action is the apparent stabilization of the balance of melatonin (diurnal stimulation) and serotonin (daylight stimulation). (37) (38)

Sound

Each body tissue resonates at a particular frequency. Both environment and disease cause variations. Vibrational medicine imparts energy to these tissues, which may bring about correctional realignments. Though scientific correlations of sound resonations and exact tissue results is lacking, therapeutic ultrasound for drug delivery systems across the skin, into tumors, into blood clots, and for physical therapy have been verified. Ultrasound therapy was used with medications in the combined treatment of primary open-angle glaucoma with promising results. The mechanism of action was proposed to be on the ocular hemodynamics of the trabecular meshwork. (39) (40)

Magnetic Therapy

No positive effects on health and healing have been established conclusively with evidence-based studies. Though hemoglobin is weakly magnetic, it appears that the fields used for calculation were too weak to give a measureable effect on either blood flow or oxygenation. MRI studies show no effects of electromagnetic therapy on bone, organs, or muscle tissue. (41) (42) Studies were negative for treating pain with magnets, but weakly positive for relief of osteoarthritis. The proposed mechanism is through stimulation of the flow of positive and negative particles in blood, fluid spaces and tissues; some neurons may be depolarized and others activated resulting in a change in action potentials. It is not clear whether this response is due to placebo or magnetic effect. (43) (44) (45) (46) Since magnetism is easily detected by the subjects, randomized, placebo-controlled trials are inconclusive and difficult to mask.

In bioelectromagnetics, the response of body tissues to electromagnetic fields produced by low-frequency pulses was generally positive in cases of multiple sclerosis, fibromyalgia, skin ulcer healing, knee joint osteoarthritis, and pain perception. Though conclusive evidence was insufficient, enough positive therapeutic effects were recorded to warrant further scientific investigation. (47) Studies showed that blood viscosity was significantly reduced with magnetic field pulsing, which may be beneficial in cardiovascular and ocular conditions that are dependent on regular blood flow. (48)

Though definitive damage to the nervous system from cell phone radiation has been scientifically refuted, many signs and symptoms are still being reported without evidence.

References for Chapter Nine:

1. Rubik B. J Altern Complement Med. 2002 Dec; 8(6): 703-17. The biofield hypothesis: Its biophysical basis and role in medicine.
2. Rindfleisch JA. Prim Carc. 2010 Mar: 37(1): 165-79. Biofield therapies: energy medicine and primary care.
3. Sicher F, et al. West J Med. 1998 Dec; 169(6): 356-63. A randomized double-blind study of the effect of distant healing in a population with advanced AIDS. Report of a small scale study.
4. Astin JA, et al. Alterm Ther Health Med. 2006 Nov-Dec; 12(6): 36-41. The efficacy of dictant healing for human immunodeficiency virus—results of a randomized trial.
5. Carvalho PA, et al. Oral Oncol. 2011 Sep 10. Evaluation of low-level laser therapy in the prevention and treatment of radiation-induced mucositis: A double-blind randomized study in head and neck cancer patients.
6. Lee WW, et al. Ophthal Plast Reconstr Surg. 2011 Jul-Aug; 27(4): 263-5. Ocular damage secondary to intense pulse light therapy to the face.
7. Kakigi R, Shibaski H. J Neurol Neurosurg Psychiatry. 1992 Apr; 55(4): 282-6. Mechanisms of pain relief by vibration and movement.
8. So PS, Jiang Y, Qin Y. Cochrane database Syst Rev. 2008 Oct 8; (4): CD006535. Touch therapies for pain relief in adults.
9. Luo DG, et al. Science. 2011 Jun 10: 332(6035): 1307-12. Activation of visual pigments by light and heat.
10. Diffey BL, Phys. Med Biol. 25; (3) Ultraviolet radiation physics and the skin.
11. Paul MA, et al. Aviat Space Environ Med. 2007 Jul; 76(7): 645-52. Circadian phase delay induced by phototherapeutic devices.
12. Gooley JJ, et al. Sci Transl Med. 2010 May 12; 2(31): 31. Spectral responses of human circadian system depend on the irradiance and duration of exposure to light.
13. Brown GM, et al. Travel Med Infect Dis. 2009 Mar; 7(2): 69-81. Melatonin and its relevance to jet lag.

14. Cajochen C, et al. J Appl Physiol. 2011 May; 110(5): 1432-8. Evening exposure to a light-emitting diodes (LED)-backlit computer screen affects circadian physiology and cognitive performance.
15. Shin HS, et al. Comp Biochem Physiol A Mol Integr Physiol. 2011 Oct; 160(2): 221-8. Effects of LED light spectra on oxidative stress and the protective role of melatonin in relation to the daily rhythm of the yellowtail clownfish, Amphiprion clarkia.
16. Tuunainen A, et al. Cochrane Database Syst Rev. 2004;(2): CD004050. Light therapy for non-seasonal depression.
17. Terman M, Terman JS. CNS Spectr. 2005 Aug; 10(8): 647-63. Light therapy for seasonal and non-seasonal depression: efficacy, protocol, safety, and side effects.
18. Benedetti F, et al. J Clin Psychiatry. 2003 Jun; 64(6): 648-53. Morning light treatment hastens the antidepressant effect of citalopram: a placebo-controlled trial.
19. Vinck EM, et al. Photomed Laser Surg. 2005 Apr; 23(2): 167-71. Green light emitting diode irradiation enhances fibroblast growth impaired by high glucose level.
20. Vinck EM, et al. Lasers Med Sci. 2003; 18(2): 95-9. Increased fibroblast proliferation induced by light emitting diode and low power laser irradiation.
21. Whelan HT, et al. J Clin Laser Med Surg. 2001 Dec: 19(6): 305-14. Effect of NASA light-emitting diode irradiation on wound healing.
22. Skopin MD, Molitor SC. Photodermatol Photoimmunol Photomed. 2009 Apr; 25(2): 75-80 Effects of near-infrared laser exposure in a cellular model of wound healing.
23. Posten W, et al. Dermatol surg. 2005 Mar; 31(3): 334-40. Low-level laser therapy for wound healing: mechanism and efficacy.
24. Tan KL. Ann Acad Med Singapore. 1993 Mar; 22(2): 225-8. Neonatal jaundice: update on phototherapy management
25. Csoma Z, Kemeny L, Olah J. N Engl J Med. 2008 Jun 5; 358(23): 2523-4. Phototherapy for neonatal jaundice.

26. Willis GL, Turner EJ. Chronobiol Int. 2007; 24(3): 521-37. Primary and secondary features of Parkinson's disease improve with strategic exposure to bright light: a case study.
27. Paus S, et al. Mov Disord. 2007 Jul 30; 22(10): 1495-8. Bright light therapy in Parkinson's disease: a pilot study.
28. Kürzinger GR, et al. Klin Monbi Augenheilkd. 2010 Jun; 227(6): 501-6. [Photodynamic therapy with verteporfin in occult choroidal neovascularization in age-related macular degeneration].
29. Lucas RM. Eye Contact Lens. 2011 Jul;37(4): 168-75. An epidemiological perspective of ultraviolet exposure—public health concerns.
30. Green AC, et al. Prog Biophys Mol Biol. 2011 Sep 3.Childhood exposure to ultraviolet radiation and harmful skin effects: Epidemiological evidence.
31. Mroz P, et al. PLos One. 2010 Dec 14; 5(12):e15194.Photodynamic therapy of tumors can lead to development of systemic antigen-specific immune response.
32. Wolffsohn JS, et al. Ophthalmic Physiol Opt. 2002 Jul; 22(4): 300-11. Benefit of coloured lenses for age-related macular degeneration.
33. Carruthers HR, et al. BMC Complement Altern Med. 2010 Dec 7; 10: 75. Mood color choice helps to predict response to hypnotherapy in patients with irritable bowel sundrome.
34. Meesters Y, et al. BMC Psychiatry. 2011 Jan 28; 11: 17. Low-intensity blue-enriched white light (750 lux) and standard bright light (10,000 lux) are equally effective in treating SAD. A randomized controlled study.
35. Vidal-López J. Percept Mot Skills. 2011 Jun; 112(3): 770-82. The role of attributional bias and visual stress on the improvement of reading speed using colored filters.
36. Dijkstra K, et al. J Adv Nurs. 2006 Oct; 56(2): 166-81. Physical environmental stimuli that turn healthcare facilities into healing environments through psychologically mediated effects: systematic review.

37. Vojnkovic B, et al. Coll Antropol. 2010 Apr; 34 Suppl 2: 89-93. Chromotherapy of macular degeneration with transitions lenses and green-yellow medical filters and special programme for psychoorganic disturbances.
38. Wolffsohn JS, et al. Ophthalmic Physiol Opt. 2002 Jul; 22(4): 300-11. Benefit of coloured lenses for age-related macular degeneration.
39. Mitragotri S. Nat Rev Drug Discov. 2005 Mar; 4(3): 255-60. Healing sound: the use of ultrasound in drug delivery and other therapeutic applications.
40. Novikova EG, Baranov VI. Vopr Kurortol Fizioter Lech Fiz Kult. 2010 Sep-Oct; (5): 33-5. [The use of biologically controlled ultrasound therapy for the combined treatment of primary open-angle glaucoma].
41. Johansesn C. Scand J Work Environ Health. 2004; 30 Suppl 1: 1-30. Electromagnetic fields and health effects—epidemiologic studies of cancer, diseases of the central nervous system and arrhythmia-related heart disease.
42. Kwon MS, et al. Bioelectromagnetics. 2011 Sep 19. No effects of short-term GSM mobile phone radiation on cerebral blood flow measured using positron emission tomography.
43. Pitter MH, Brown EM, Ernst E. CMAJ. 2007 Sep 25; 177(7): 736-42. Static magnets for reducing pain: systematic review and meta-analysis of randomized trials.
44. Harlow T, et al. BMJ. 2004 Dec 18; 329(7480): 1450-4. Randomized controlled trial of magnetic bracelets for relieving pain in osteoarthritis of the hip and knee.
45. McCarthy CJ, et al. BMC Musculoskeletal Disord. 2006 Jun 15; 7: 51. Pulsed electromagnetic energy treatment offers no clinical benefit in reducing the pain of knee osteoarthritis: a systematic review.
46. Richmond SJ, et al. Complement Ther Med. 2009 Oct-Dec; 17(5-6): 249-56. Therapeutic effects of magnetic and copper bracelets in osteoarthritis: a randomized placebo-controlled crossover trial.

47. Therapeutic effects of whole-body devices applying pulsed electromagnetic fields (PEMF): A systematic literature review. [No authors]
48. Tao R, Huang K. Phys Rev E Stat Nonlin Soft Matter Phys. 2011 Jul; 84(1-1):011905 Reducing blood viscosity with magnetic fields.

Traditional Chinese and Ayurvedic Medicine and the Eyes

Case Scenario One: Mrs. B is an open-minded 68-year-old patient of Dr. A. She has just been diagnosed with age-related macular degeneration and borderline glaucoma. Both of her elderly parents were debilitated from the same a.m. despite multiple interventional treatments. She has been reading about complimentary medicine and asks her doctor about available treatment options other than anti-VEGF, PDT, and laser surgery. She asks about the expected prognosis and risks associated with treatments like acupuncture, herbs and dietary supplements. Dr. A is also open-minded and well-acquainted with complementary medical treatments. He provides her with enough information to enable her to make a decision on a reasonable plan for her treatment.

Acupuncture (pain relief)	Moxibustion (dry eyes)	Chinese & Ayurvedic herbs
Eastern diet (antioxidants)	Yoga	Eye exercises

Table 1: Eastern Medicine and the Eyes:

Pain relief	Dry eye syndrome	Age-related macular degeneration
Glaucoma	Cataract	Neurodegenerative diseases

Table 2. Indications for the use of Eastern Medicine:

The clinical trials and evidence-based research studies for the specific use of eastern medicine for eye conditions like myopia, strabismus, retinitis pigmentosa, optic atrophy, retrobulbar neuritis, cataract, glaucoma, maculopathies, conjunctivitis, and iritis, are limited. The suggested modalities are being included existing alternative therapies and in anticipation of further, more conclusive studies with specific positive or negative outcomes.

Caution: The use of these treatment modalities are contraindicated in cases of serious disease, bleeding tendencies, epilepsy, in patients with pacemakers, and in any case, where conventional or other alternative therapy is available.

Acupuncture has been an integral part of the Chinese health care system for 5,000 years. It is reported to correct the imbalance of energy flow (chi) along specific channels (meridians) throughout the body. Skin stimulation with needles releases opioid peptides and endorphins known as enkephalins. These provide analgesia by affecting the small *C* fibers, carrying pain impulses in response to excess stimulation, regulating the secretion of the neurotransmitters, serotonin and norepinephrine, directly stimulating the end-organ nerve pathways and inhibiting prostacyclins and thromboxane pain factors. This analgesia is reproducible in double-blind studies in both humans and animals in the laboratory. Acupuncture has a direct effect on immunity by raising levels of triglycerides, prostaglandins, gamma globulins, and white blood cells, and also by releasing histamines. (1) (2)

Acupuncture for glaucoma produced an improvement in central visual acuity but no change in intraocular pressure or visual fields. (3) The Cochrane Eyes and Vision Group US project reported in 2007 that there were no randomized clinical trials and limited evidence for its use in established glaucoma. (4)

Acupuncture for age-related macular degeneration was found to have more positive effects than intramuscular Entodon, and oral vitamin C and E. In 2003, the American Academy of Ophthalmology (AAO) issued a statement to the effect that there was insufficient evidence to demonstrate the safety or effectiveness of acupuncture for age-related macular degeneration. It was also suggested that even though there was a tendency toward the relief of dry eyes, migraine and tension headache with needle acupuncture, a determination of efficacy and justification for routine use could not be established. Acupuncture has been used successfully to provide anesthesia for strabismus surgery. (5) (6)

Moxibustion and lacrimal massage for dry eyes was found to have a positive therapeutic effect through tears secretion testing, lacrimal membrane breaking time, and corneal fluorescent staining before and after treatment. But there was insufficient evidence to warrant its use over conventional therapies. (7) (8)

A positive effect in the form of a subjunctive improvement in visual acuity from acupuncture on myopia, glaucoma, retinitis pigmentosa, and optic nerve atrophy together, with a positive observation by visual field perimetry, light sensitivity, and electrooculograms have been reported but the methods and conclusions are deemed insufficient for evidence-based medicine. (9)

The doctor may instruct the patient that though an AAO task force reported that acupuncture may be useful as adjunctive therapy and is an acceptable alternative to conventional medicine, it would not be a first line of therapy. (10) By releasing blockage and accumulation of toxins, acupuncture works for removing excesses. Chinese and Ayurvedic herbs, and heat are more suited for building up deficiencies.

Cataracts:	Chrysanthemum flowers	Zhang-Yan-Ming	Pa-Wei-Di Huan-Wan	Triphala
Inflammation:	Gentian	Celosia seeds	Buddleia	Pagoda tree
Circulation:	Red sage	Ginkgo biloba	Motherwort	Angelica
Immunity:	Astragalus	Schisandra	Cordyceps	Triphala
Dry eyes:	Dendrobium			
ARMD:	Wolfberry (goji)			

Table 3: Chinese and Ayurvedic Herbals for the Eyes*

**The herbs listed are but a few representing the vast materia medica of Chinese herbal medicine that are associated with health of the eyes.*

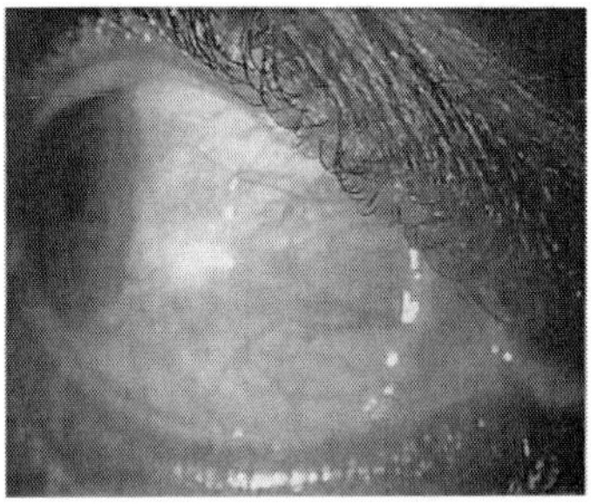

inflammation

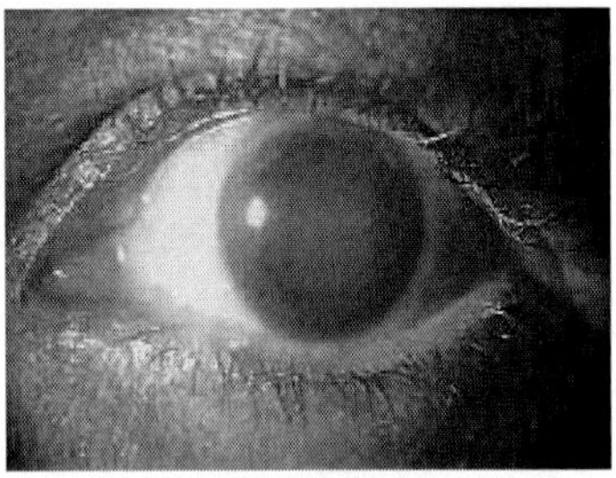

nuclear cataract

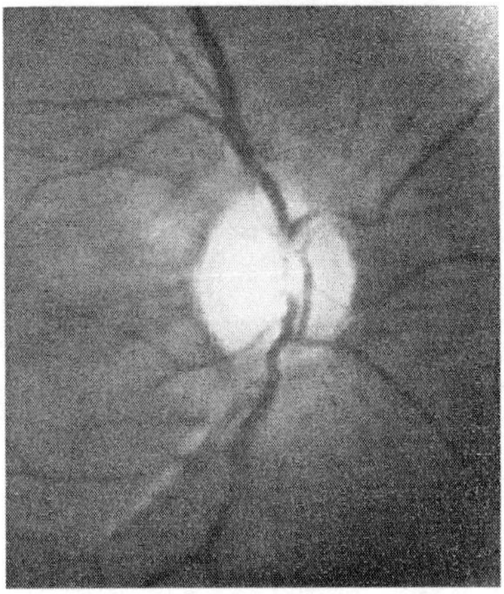

poor circulation

The intricate combinations of Chinese herbs are designed to influence the factors causing diseases especially in relation to the aging process, toxic effects of smoking, ultraviolet radiation, topical and systemic steroids, trauma, diabetic sorbitol excess, hereditary protein irregularities, adverse medications, and an antioxidant-deficient diet.

Chrysanthemum flowers (Ju Hua) cultivated in China, contain two flavones glycosides, which were found to reduce cataract formation by inhibiting the activity of rat lens aldose reductase. Two separate studies isolated components with the similar inhibitory activity. (11) (12) In Chinese medicine, disorders of the liver and kidney are linked to inflammatory conditions of the eyes. Chrysanthemum has been used to alleviate these symptoms. It is taken most often in the form of a tea to which goji berries may be added for more antioxidant activity.

Zhang-Yin-Ming and *Pa Wei Di Huang Wan* are two Chinese herbals effective in inhibiting the formation of sorbitol in the crystalline lens due to their flavonoid content and strong antioxidant activity. (13)

Triphala is an Ayurvedic combination of three fruits, *Emblica officinalis*, *Terminalia chebula,* and *Terminalia bellirica*, which has been found to retard the development of selenite-induced cataracts in rats in both in vitro and in vivo studies. Its activity is attributed to its high antioxidant content, which restores and maintains the actions of enzymes like superoxide dismutase, glutathione peroxidase, catalase, and glutathione-s-transferase. (14)

Other herbals with anticataract activity (for which sufficient experimental data could not be found) include celosia seeds (Qing xiang zi) and plantago seeds (Che qian zi).

Chinese Gentian (*Gentiana sino-ornata*) (Lung-tan Tsao) is a bitter herb, which, when taken orally, has been found to cleanse the liver, benefit digestion, and general body weakness. Its active ingredients include terpenoids and geraniol, which are anti-inflammatory and anti-irritative. It has been used to relieve acute conjunctivitis and jaundice. (15)

Active ingredients from the seeds of the flowering plant, *Celosia argentea,* consist of celogentin peptides with antimitotic activity that has been shown to have liver restorative activities, which result in improvement of red, painful, inflamed eyes. (16)

Buddleia flower bud and pagoda tree flowers are also used traditionally to treat red eyes and failing eyesight from liver inflammation, but evidence-based studies were not readily available.

Red sage (danshen) root proved best at resisting blood stasis induced by dextran and in promoting blood circulation in experimental groups of rabbits. (17)

Ginkgo biloba extract was found to be effective with statistically significant improvements in distance visual acuity in a double-blind, placebo study in a small population. The mechanism of action was by inhibition of clotting with improved status of the macular degeneration. (18) A Cochrane database study revealed that though a beneficial effect was observed, the consumption of *Ginkgo biloba* extract did not slow or prevent the progression of age-related macular degeneration. (19) Caution should be used when using ginkgo with aspirin as both are blood thinners and have been cited for pupillary margin hemorrhage and potential retinal bleeding especially in diabetics. (20)

An extract of the dried aerial parts of Chinese motherwort (*Leonurus heterophyllus*) was shown to promote blood circulation and reduce blood stasis through its inhibition of tissue factor expression. It also has anticancer activity. (21)

Angelica sinensis root (dong quai) is used in Chinese medicine to enrich the blood, promote circulation, and regulate the immune system through its antioxidant activity. It also affects the eyes through its neuro- and hepatoprotective activities. (22) (23)

Many diseases of the eyes progress rapidly when the immune system of the organism is compromised. A healthy immune system with a well-regulated response is essential to good functioning of the ocular tissues.

The bark of the astragalus (*A. villosus*) (Huang qi) plant shows positive immunological activity through its high content of polysaccharides. Testing on the immune response to foot-and-mouth disease virus (FMDV) induced in pigs resulted in a marked increase in FMDV-specific antibodies. It may be taken routinely with excellent safety and efficacy and is especially beneficial in older age groups with waning immunity function. (24) (25)

Extracts from the fruit of *Schisandra chinensis* (wu wei zi) show strong immune-regulatory properties and has been used traditionally to treat general fatigue, neurasthenia, and diaphoresis. Its mechanism of action is via the increased release of cytokines by THP-1 cells in promoting cell-mediated and humoral immunity when challenged by antigenic stimulation. One of its components, Schisandrin C, along with two other lignans, gomisin J and N, has been shown to reduce the process of lipopolysaccharide-induced inflammation by reducing the expression of mRNA and the secretion of proinflammatory cytokines. (26) (27)

Cordyceps sinensis is a Chinese mushroom, which acts as an immune system suppressor much in a similar way as prednisone. Studies have shown it to be significantly safer than corticosteroids with respect to side effects and organ damage. It can be used in transplant cases where treatment with prednisone is contraindicated or has exhibited an over response. It also shows a strong inhibition of lipid peroxidation through the strong antioxidant activity of its polysaccharides. (28) (29)

Triphala may be used topically and systemically to treat immune modulated inflammatory responses from oxidative stress, excitatory infectious disease neutrophils, excess radiation, and arthritis inflammation. One teaspoon of powder in water, left overnight, strained, and liquid applied to the eyes for several days, will reduce the symptoms. (30) 31) (32)

A combination of extracts of *Dendrobium* flowers with *Chrysanthemum*, wolfberry, *Rehmannia*, figwort, lilyturf root, and sticktight, taken orally along with a tear film lubricant, has been shown to reduce the symptoms of dry eyes in postmenopausal women better than with the tear film lubricant alone. The active ingredients of dendrobium have been credited with promoting the aqueous aspect of tear secretion. (33)

In a well-constructed double-masked, randomized, placebo-controlled study, the daily dietary supplementation with wolfberry (goji berry) (*Lycium barbarum*) (Gou Qi Zi) for a period of thirty days increased the antioxidant efficacies in humans by stimulating endogenous factors regulating lipid peroxidaton, and serum levels of glutasthione peroxidase and superoxide dismutase. Its active properties are attributed to high polysaccharide levels, which may act to prevent or lessen free radical-related conditions. (34) A similar study confirmed the protective positive antioxidant effect of *Lycium barbarum* polysaccharides in aged mice. (35)

Another Chinese herb, pseudoginseng root (san qi) has been purported to stop eye bleeding, but no evidence-based studies could be found.

Chinese medicine treats eye disease largely by addressing the disorders of liver and kidney. Conjunctivitis, asthenopia, and inflammations like prostatis and urinary tract infections are attributed to excess liver heat. Failing eyesight due to aging is due to kidney dysfunction. Basic restorative nutritional practices consisting of warming and cooling foods have been shown to assist with healing of these organs and subsequent improvement in vision and relief of symptoms.

Chinese and Ayurvedic Eye exercises:

The prevalence of high myopia in Asian populations are well documented. (36) Regular eye exercises have been promoted in school-aged children to improve eyesight, though clearly outlined clinical studies are limited. Moving the eyes in the four basic directions of gaze (right, left, up, and down) and then rotating them clockwise and counterclockwise, is a simple exercise. This maintains the muscles and affects fixation and gaze, but lends questionable improvement to visual acuity. The action of palming may be used to rest the eyes and is purported to improve amblyopia and relief stress. The palms of both hands are rubbed together for about thirty seconds and applied gently to the closed lids. The warmth may stimulate blood flow through small-vessel dilation. Which vessels are affected and how effective the method is could not be identified in the literature. Relief of eyestrain during study periods, and TV and computer use is effectively reduced by avoidance. Massaging specific areas around the eye (Zan zhu, Shibai, and Taiyang points) are purported to offer relief as well.

Yoga for strengthening the eye muscles is done in a seated, poised position (Sukhasana) and moving the eyes in four gaze positions and clockwise and counterclockwise, with intervals of lid closure. The practice of yoga was reported to reduce the symptoms of vision discomfort in a group of computer users more than a similar group who did not use yoga. (37)

Caution: Possible contraindications to practicing yoga should be considered since several adverse events like central retinal vein occlusion and progressive optic neuropathy in congenital glaucoma have been associated with the headstand position (Sirsasana). (38) (39)

The Ayurvedic diet is rich in antioxidant fruit and vegetables and herbs for the maintenance of general health, which affects the eyes and other senses and intends to realign the natural energy of the body (prana) for purposes of proper functioning. It is directed primarily towards the regulation of the musculoskeletal and nervous systems. Characteristics of the Vata dosha, which is associated with movement of the body and nervous system activities, are particularly attached to the eyes. The application of cooling water to eyes in the morning, warm water to feet in the evening, and the drinking of fennel seeds water for eye lubrication is said to contribute to good eye health. The Pitta dosha, which controls digestion, metabolism, and energy production, is concentrated on reducing stress, eye tension, and redness from grief, anger, and worry. Cellular and tissue growth, body structure, and fluid balance are attributed to the Kapha dosha. Adequate evidence-based research studies for their functions and effects are limited.

References for Chapter Ten:

1. NIH consensus conference. Acupuncture. JAMA, 1998; 280: 1518-24.
2. Leake R, Broderick JE. Integrative Medicine 1998; 1: 107-15. Treatment efficacy of acupuncture: a review of the research literature.
3. Rhee DJ, et al. Surv Ophthalmol. 2001 Jul-Aug; 46(1): 43-55. Complementary and alternative medicine for glaucoma.
4. Law SK, Tianjing L. Cochrane Eyes and Vision Group US Project, Baltimore, USA. Acupuncture for glaucoma.
5. Jiao NJ. Zhongguo Zhen Jiu. 2011 Jan; 31(1):43-5. [Observation on therapeutic effect of age-related macular degeneration treated with acupuncture].
6. American Academy of Ophthalmology Complementary Therapy Assessment: acupuncture for ocular conditions and headaches. AAO,May 2003.
7. Chen LQ. Zhongguo Zhen Jiu. 2008 Aug:28(8):585-8. [Observation on therapeutic effect of moxibustion with thunder-fire herbal moxa stick on xerophthalmia of oligodacrya].
8. Halevi S. Journal of Chinese Medicine in England. Acupuncture. com 2000. Acupuncture and snail shell moxibustioon in the treatment of eye diseases. Pt II.
9. Dabor S, et al. Acupuncture Electrother Res. 1985; 10(1-2): 79-93. Clinical application of acupuncture in ophthalmology.

10. American Academy of Ophthalmology Complementary Therapy Assessment: acupuncture for ocular conditions and headaches. San Francisco: AAO, 1999.
11. L. Yoshokawa M, et al. Chem Pharm Bull (Tokyo). 1999 Mar; 47(3): 340-5. Medicinal flowers I. Aldose reductase inhibitors and three new eudesmane-type sesquiterpenes, Kikkanols A, B, and C, from flowers of Chrysanthemum indicum
12. Matsuda H, et al. Chem Pharm Bull (Tokyo). 2002 Jul; 50(7): 972-5. Medicinal flowers VI. Absolute stereostructures of two new flavones glycosides and a phenyl butanoid glycoside from the flowers of Chrysanthemum indicum L.: their inhibitory activities for rat lens aldose reductase.
13. Chiou GC, et al. J Ocul Pharmacol. 1992 Summer; 8(2): 115-20. Effects of some natural products on sugar cataract studied with nuclear magnetic resonance spectroscopy.
14. Gupta SK, et al. J Ayurveda Integr Med. 2010 Oct-Dec; 1(4): 280-286. Evaluation of anticataract potential of Triphala in selenite-induced cataract: In vitro and in vivo studies.
15. Thoppil RJ, Bishayee A. World J Hepatol. 2011 September 27; 3(9): 228-249. Terpenoids as potential chemopreventive and therapeutic agents in liver cancer.
16. Ma B, et al. J Am Chem Soc. 2010. Jan 27; 132(3): 1159-1171. Total Synthesis of the Antimitotic Bicyclic Peptide Celogentin C.
17. Lu Y, et al. J Ethnopharmacol. 2008 Mar 5; 116(2): 313-7. Selection of component drug in activating blood flow and removing blood stasis of Chinese herbal medicinal formula for dairy cow mastitis by hemorrheological method.
18. LeBuisson DA, et al. Presse Med. 1986 Sept 25; 15(31): 1556-8. [Treatment of senile macular degeneration with ginkgo biloba extract: a preliminary double-blind drug vs placebo study].
19. Evans JR. Cochrane Database Syst Rev. 2000; (2): CD001775. Ginkgo biloba extract for age-related macular degeneration.

20. N Engl J Med 1997; 336:1108. Spontaneous hyphaema associated with ingestion of Ginkgo biloba extract.
21. Yin J, et al. Am J Chin Med. 2010 ; 38(1):157-71.Stachydrine, a major constituent of the Chinese herb Leonurus heterophyllus sweet, ameliorates human umbilical vein endothelial cells injury induced by anoxia-reoxygenation.
22. Wu YC, Hsieh CL. Chin Med. 2011 Aug 25; 6: 32. Pharmacological effects of Radix Angelica Sinensis (Danggui) on cerebral infarction.
23. Chao WW, Lin BF. Chin Med. 2011 Aug 19; 6:29. Bioactivities of major constituents isolated from Angelica sinensis (Danggui),
24. Block KL, Mead MN. Integr Cancer Ther. 2003 Sep; 2(3): 247-67. Immune system effects of Echinacea, ginseng and astragalus: a review.
25. Li J, et al. Int J Biol Macromol. 2011 Oct 1; 49(3): 362-8. Enhancement of Astragalus polysaccharides on the immune responses in pigs inoculated with foot-and-mouth disease virus vaccine
26. Lin RD, et al. Molecules. 2011 Jun 10; 16(6):4836-49. The immune-regulatory effects of Schisandra chinensis and its constituents on human monocytic leukemia cells.
27. Oh SY, et al. Biosci Biotechnol Biochem. 2010; 74(2): 285-91. Anti-inflammatory effects of gomisin N, gomisin J, and schisandrin C isolated from the fruit of Schisandra chinensis.
28. Li SP. Et al. Phytomedicine. 2001 May; 8(3): 207-12. Anti-oxidation activity of different types of natural Cordyseps sinensis and cultured Cordyseps mycelia.
29. Ding CG, et al. Zhongguo Zhong Xi Yi Jie He Za Zhi. 2009 Nov; 29(11): 975-8. [Clinical application and exploration on mechanism of action of Cordyseps sinensis mycella preparation for renal transplantation recipients.
30. SriKuma R, et al. Biol Pharm Bull. 2005 Aug; 28(8):1398-403. Immunomodulatory activity of triphala in neutrophil functions.
31. Sandhya T, et al. Mutat Res. 2006 Oct 10; 609(1): 17-25. Protection against radiation oxidative damage in mice by Triphala.

32. Rasool M, Sabina EP. Phytother Res. 2007 Sep; 21(9): 889-94. Anti inflammatory effect of the Indian Ayurvedic herbal formulation Triphala on adjuvant-induced arthritis in mice.
33. Wei D, Li YH, Zhou WY. Zhongguo Zhong Xi Yi Jie He Za Zhi. 2009 Jul; 29(7): 646-9. [Observation on Therapeutic effect of runmushu oral liquid in treating xerophthalmia in postmenopausal women].
34. Buchell P, et al. Optom Vis Sci. 2011 Feb; 88(2): 257-62. Goji berry effects on macular characteristics and plasma antioxidant levels.
35. Amagase H, Sun B, Borek C. Nutr Res. 2009 Jan; 29(1):19-25. Lycium barbarum (goji) juice improves in vivi antioxidant biomarkers in serum of healthy adults.
36. Li XM, Ma YL, Liu XJ. J Ethnopharmacol. 2007 May 22; 111(3):504-11. Effect of Lycium barbarum polysaccharides on age-related oxidative stress in aged mice.
37. Tan CS, et al. Eye (Lond). 2011 Oct; 25(10): 294-301. Prevalence and risk factors for refractive errors and ocular biometry parameters in an elderly Asian population: The Singapore Longitudinal Aging Study (SLAS).
38. Telles S, et al. Head Face Med. 2006 Dec 3; 2:46. Effect of yoga on self-rated visual discomfort in computer users.
39. deBarrios DS, et al. Ophthalmic surg Lasers Imaging. 2008 Jul-Aug; 39(4): 339-40. Progressive optic neuropathy in congenital glaucoma associated with the Sirsasana yoga posture.
40. Shah NJ, Shah UN. Indian J Ophthalmol. 2009 Jan-Feb; 57(1): 68-70. Central retinal vein occlusion following Sirsasana (headstand posture).

Homeopathy for the Eyes

Case Scenario One: I have recurrent redness of the eyes and they feel tired and painful. I tried a lot of medications, but they only make it worse. Can homeopathic medicines possibly help my eyes? And how do they work?

Homeopathy is a form of complementary medicine in which highly diluted preparations of substances that may cause symptoms in healthy people are used to treat similar symptoms in the patient. Known as "The law of Similars," the basic principle is to "let like be cured by like." Developed in 1796 by the German physician, Samuel Hahnemann, the principles of homeopathy have not been proven by scientific method, but its positive results have been compared to those of the placebo effect. (1) The placebo effect works, is safe, cheap, proven, and well researched. The idea of treatment acts to elicit a positive reaction via psychological or biochemical responses with endorphins as the effective vehicles. Homeopathy works, but not by the rules of conventional medicine. Some argue that since pharmacological effects and dose-responsive relationships are not reproducible based on a miniscule amount of active chemical substance, studies in homeopathy are not worthwhile. Since it does work, attention should be given to the paradigm at times to include anecdotal and observational evidence. (2)

Nevertheless, conventional medical journals continue to downplay the positive effects of homeopathic remedies while stressing the limits and lack of reproducibility, while alternative medical journals report the positive aspects of research studies. (3)

The advice to the patient can be simplified into "Yes, it works," but not by scientific method. Low dilutions appear to work like vaccinations and so are favored by conventional medicine while higher dilutions contain little or no substance, and work by vital force and energy as postulated by the core principles of homeopathy. Possible mechanisms of action include the range of mobilizing the body's defenses to stimulate the healing responses and act against the disease to the very intricacies of cellular entanglement in quantum physics. However simple and complicated at the same time, it appears to work in some cases. (4) (5)

Caution: Since homeopathic remedies are recommended to be taken alone, care must be used that they should not take the place of conventional treatments when serious diseases are being addressed. To avoid inducing infections, only the best preparations from reputable companies should be used.

Traumatic Ecchymosis	Blepharitis	Conjunctivitis with discharge	Conjunctivitis with red eyes, lesion, foregn body
Corneal ulcer	Cataract	Glaucoma (acute)	Iritis with intraocular inflammation
Chorioretinitis	Retinal hemorrhage	Retinitis pigmentosa	Asthenopia with eyestrain

Table 1. Indications for Homeopathic Treatment for the Eyes

Many eye conditions can be made worse by the application of conventional pharmaceutical eyedrops and ointments that contain hyperallergenic vehicles, like benzalkonium chloride, which induce congestion and hyperemia. Some patients simply cannot afford strong conventional drugs and office visits. For these cases, homeopathic remedies could be a consideration.

Homeopathic medicines for eye conditions are substances that would induce the same symptoms in the eyes for which they are being treated. When derived from diseased or pathological products, like fecal matter, discharge, blood, or tissue, the treatments are called *nosodes*. When prepared from healthy specimens, like plants and minerals, they are called *sarcodes*. When compared directly with anti-inflammatory conventional medications (indomethacin versus a combination of apis, lachesis, arnica, belladonna, hamamelis, and phosphorus), the homeopathic route showed a statistical significant reduction in edema in the rat model in the first phase of testing but did not hold up as well in the second phase. (6) In modern medicine, homeopathy should not be ignored and discarded but should be addressed through more and better study designs.

Most homeopathic remedies may be taken two to three times daily in small pill form, dissolvable under the tongue and for four to five days depending on the severity of symptoms. Many of the following homeopathic remedies for eyes have undergone scientific evaluation and will be so indicated. There have been no side effects reported.

Aconite	Allium cepa	Arnica	Belladonna	Bryonia
Causticum/ Casticum	Silicea/Coniu m	Calcarea flourica	Euphrasia	Ferrum phosphoricum
Gelsemium	Hamamelis	Kalium bichromicum	Kalium muriaticum	Kalium sulphuricum
Lachesis and Crotalus	Ledum	Mercurius vivus	Natrum muriaticum	Opium/cocaine muriate, spigella
Phosphorus	Pulsatilla	Rhus toxicodendron	Ruta graveolens	Sabadilla

Table 2. Homeopathic Treatment for the Eyes

Ledum is derived from the wild rosemary plant and is used in cases of traumatic ecchymosis and puncture wounds of the lids due to animal and insect bites.

Pulsatilla (*P. nigricans*) from the pasque flower plant causes profuse lachrymation and meibomian gland agglutination of secretions in healthy eyes. When used early in the treatment of styes, it may prevent the formation of pus. It is also used in cases of conjunctivitis with profuse green discharge.

Aconite is used for early conjunctivitis from trauma, foreign body, photophobia, and painful acute superficial inflammation, associated with wounds and burns.

Rhus toxicodendron is used to treat conjunctival chemosis with discharge as occurs with exposure to poisonous plants. It must be noted that cases of orbital cellulitis can be life threatening and are more wisely treated with conventional medicines first, and with homeopathics only as last resort. Droopy eyelids after cataract surgery with impending iritis and rheumatic ptosis also have been observed to respond to this homeopathic treatment. (7)

Allium cepa is a diluted form of onions used as a remedy for excessive tearing and itching of the eyes. Onion juice applied to rats' eyes with selenite-induced cataracts showed a reduction in formation of the lesions. (8)

In one study, extracts of arnica (and stinging nettle) were found to be more successful in reducing the pain of erbium-YAG laser-induced burns than placebos. These can be applied to abrasions of the eyelids and the periorbital area. In a review of eight trials using *Arnica montana* for relief of tissue trauma, efficacy beyond that of placebo was not supported, though methodological flaws were noted in most. (9) (10) *Arnica montana* and *Bryonia* were administered orally after aortic valve surgery for control of pain and inflammation and found to offer no statistical difference from placebo. (11)

Belladonna (*Atropa belladonna)* is the frequently used homeopathic remedy for eye troubles and is indicated for sudden acute inflammation, dry, injected eyes, absence of tears, as in acute conjunctivitis, iritis, retinitis, with pronounced photophobia and dilated pupils. Though a randomized, double-blind, placebo-controlled proving trials reported no observable clinical effects, a second report on the same trials disputed the conclusion. (12) (13) When a 30H dilution of belladonna was tested for the production of symptoms as compared to placebo and observation, there was no significant difference. (14)

Euphrasia (*E. officinalis*) is used as an eyewash for persistent lid inflammation, conjunctivitis, corneal ulcers from trauma, and excessive tearing associated with allergies,

Ferrum phosphoricum, mercurius and sabadilla (*Asagrea officinalis*) can be used for the early stages of acute catarrh with burning, red, congested eyes, and absent discharge.

Kalium bichromicum, a potassium compound, is used to treat inflammation associated with corneal ulcers with tendency to perforate, circumscribed with clear-cut edges, and indolent eyelids. Kalium muriaticum is used for corneal inflammation and ulceration, which is chronic and without conjunctival redness, tearing or pain. Kalium sulphuricum is used for ophthalmia neonatorum, gonorrheal ophthalmias, and corneal abscess. No evidence-based efficacious studies could be found.

When a 30C dilution of natrum muriaticum and arsenicum album were tested in healthy volunteers for production of symptoms, both homeopathic remedies produced different symptoms than placebo. Natrum muriaticum, whose main ingredient is sodium chloride, can be used for conjunctival congestion and mild corneal edema as occurs in the common cold, as an eyewash in much the same way as normal saline irrigation. (15) (16)

The group of Causticum 6X HPUS, Silicea 9X, Calcarea fluorica 10X, Conium, and

Casticum have been designated as preventives of cataract formation. Their common ingredient in calcium has been implicated in cataractogenesis associated with the activation of calpain and subsequent proteolysis leading to opacification of the lens. (17)

Gelsemium sempervirens (yellow jasmine) dilates the pupil by paralyzing the oculomotor nerve. It is used to treat symptoms of diplopia, ptosis, pain, and intraocular inflammation associated with severe iritis as may occur in acute influenza. It has also been purported to relieve the pain and neurotic symptoms of glaucoma. A randomized, placebo-controlled study examining the proposed effect of gelsemium on provoked anxiety, found little or no significance. (18)

Hamamelis virginiana (witch hazel) is used for relief and healing of sore, red, painful eyes with inflamed blood vessels. It is said to hasten the absorption of hyphema.

Lachesis muta and *Crotalus horridus* are snake venoms, which are used to thin the blood, thereby inducing hemorrhage. The homeopathic preparation 200C is used to treat infection with diphtheria, after infliction with toxins and for retinal hemorrhage that does not clear with conventional prescription treatment or time, and when surgery is contraindicated or high risk.

For glaucoma, the natural heavy metal, osmium, causes increased intraocular pressure and photophobia. The eyes of individuals taking opium feel expanded, under pressure, and the pupils are constricted. Cocaine muriate, *Spigelia anthelmia*, phosphorus, and *Aconitum napellus*, give the eyes a sensation of throbbing pain and extension and the pupils are dilated as in acute angle-closure glaucoma.

Caution: This condition is best treated with immediate conventional surgery. A highly diluted preparation of phosphorus is used for retinitis pigmentosa and albuminuria, amblyopia, and asthenopia.

A homeopathic preparation of *Ruta graveolens* is used to reduce eyestrain (asthenopia) from overwork. A study to measure the antimetaplastic activity of *Ruta graveolens* and *Hydrastis canadensis* in tumor-induced rats supported the antitumor action.

Another study showed that Ruta 200C was capable of inducing genotoxicity when given at higher doses. (19) (20)

Scientific research studies with conclusions, which support homeopathic remedies that satisfy conventional medicine are limited. However, there is enough positive evidence to justify physicians being aware and having some understanding of the concept. In a study designed to observe the action of homeopathic remedies on heart rate and blood flow, sulphur, gelsemium, phosphorus and pulsatilla (all at 200C, 1M) produced a positive response in amplitude by 62 percent as compared to 16 percent with placebo. Evidence in favor of homeopathy tends to be limited because of the low-methodological quality of many trials, as if they are designed to fail. (21) (22) while homeopathy affords both pro and antisentiments, the fact remains that the good safety profile, lower costs, and moderate benefits outweigh the detractions. As long as there is a need and acceptance within the population, homeopathy should play a complementary role with conventional treatments. (23)

References for Chapter Eleven:

1. Shang, A et al (2005) The Lancet 366 (9487) 726-732. Are the clinical effects of homeopathy placebo effects? Comparative study of placebo-controlled trials of homeopathy and allopathy.
2. The National Center for Complementary and Alternative Medicine of the United States' National Institutes of Health statement: nccam.nih.gov/health/homeopathy/controversies.
3. Caulfield T, DeBow S. BMC Complement Altern Med. 2005 Jun 14; 5: 12. A systematic review of how homeopathy is represented in conventional and CAM peer reviewed journals.
4. Linde K, et al. J Clin Epidemiol. 1999 Jul; 52(7): 631-6. Impact of study quality on outcome in placebo-controlled trials of homeopathy.
5. Moiski M. Homeopathy. 2010 Apr; 99(2): 104-12. Quasi-quantum phenomena: the key to understanding homeopathy.

6. Conforti A, et al. BMC Complement Altern Med. 2007 Jan 17; 7:1. Rat models of acute inflammation: a randomized controlled study on the effects of homeopathic remedies.
7. Gladman AC. Wilderness Environ Med. 2006 Summer; 17(2): 120-8. Toxicodendron dermatitis: poison ivy, oak, and sumac.
8. Javadzadeh A, et al. Indian J Ophthalmolo. 2009 May-Jun; 57(3): 185-9. Preventive effect of onion juice on selenite-induced experimental cataract.
9. Huber R, et al. Complement Ther Med. 2011 Oct; 19(5): 276-80. Arnica and stinging nettle for treating burns- a self-experiment.
10. Ernst E, Pittler MH. Arch Surg. 1998 Nov; 133(11): 1187-90. Efficacy of homeopathic arnica: a systematic review of placebo-controlled clinical trials.
11. Cornu C, et al. Br J Clin Pharmacol. 2010 Feb; 69(2): 136-42. No effect of a homeopathic combination of Arnica Montana and Bryonia alba on bleeding, inflammation, and ischaemia after aortic valve surgery.
12. Br J Clin Pharmacol. 2003 Nov; 56(5): 562-8. Ultramolecular homeopathy has no observable clinical effects. A randomized, double-blind, placebo-controlled proving trial of Belladonna 30C.
13. Shalts E, Ahiflett S. Br J Clin Pharmacol. 2004 Sep; 58(3): 340-1. The conclusion that "ultramolecular homeopathy has no observable clinical effects" is not supported by the data.
14. Walach H, et al. J Psychosom Res. 2001 Mar; 50(3): 155-60. The effects of homeopathic belladonna 30CH in healthy volunteers- a randomized, double-blind experiment.
15. Sawyer P. Midwifery Today Int Midwife. 2003 Winter; (68): 45,67. Salt of the earth. Homeopathic Natrum muriaticum.
16. Mollinger H, Schneider R, Walach H. Forsch Komplementmed. 2009 Apr; 16(2): 105-10. Homeopathic pathogenetic trials produce specific symptoms different from placebo.
17. Lee HY, et al. Vet Ophthalmol. 2008 Nov-Dec; 11(6); 347-55. The involvement of calpains in opacification induced by Ca2+ overload in ovine lens culture.

18. Paris A, et al. Fundam Clin Pharmacol. 2011 Sep 28. Effect of Gelsemium 5CH and 15CH on anticipathy anxiety : a phase III, single-centre, randomized, placebo-controlled study.
19. Es S, et al. Asian Pac J Cancer Prev. 2007 Jul-Sep; 8(3): 390-4. Effect of homeopathic medicines on transplanted tumors in mice.
20. Preethi KC, et al. Asian Pac J Cancer Prev. 2008 Oct-Dec; 9(4): 763-9. Clastogenic potential of Ruta graveolens extract and a homeopathic preparation in mouse bone marrow cells.
21. Mishra N, et al. J Altern Complement Med. 2011 Aug; 17(8): 705-10. An exploratory study on scientific investigations in homeopathy using medical analyser.
22. Cucherat M, et al. Eur J Clin Pharmacol. 2000 Apr; 56(1): 27-33. Evidence of clinical efficacy of homeopathy. A meta-analysis of clinical trials. HMRAG. Homeopathic Medicines Research Advisory Group.
23. Ng, DY. Homeopathy. 2011 Jul; 100(3): 183-6. A discussion: the future role of homeopathy in the National Health Service (NHS).

Appendix

Aging Strategies for continued good health include adequate exercise, proper nutrition, stress control, social-spiritual-mental stimulation and avoidance of risky behavior.

General Measures For Eye Health

1. Annual eye exam over age 50.
2. Eye protection
3. Eye nutrients
4. Control of diabetes and hypertension
5. Regular exercise
6. Reduce inflammation/boost immune system

Best Herbs For Aging

1. Bilberry
2. Celery seed
3. Echinacea
4. Garlic
5. *Ginkgo biloba*
6. Hawthorn berry
7. Milk Thistle
8. St John's wort
9. Saw palmetto
10. Turmeric

Best Foods For Longevity

1. Tomatoes (lycopene)
2. Olive oil (omega-3 fatty acids)
3. Red grapes (resveratrol)
4. Garlic
5. Spinach (iron & folic acid)
6. Whole grains
7. Salmon (omega-3 fish oil)
8. Nuts & seeds
9. Blueberries (lutein & zeaxanthin)
10. Green tea (epigallocatechins)

INFLAMMATION & IMMUNITY: A dysfunctional immune system resulting in uncontrolled inflammation and delayed healing plays a major role in many eye diseases. The anti-inflammation diet includes a multivitamin (with A,C & E), omega-3 fish oil, flaxseed, garlic, ginger, turmeric, antioxidants (lutein, zeaxanthin, zinc, folic acid, selenium, Co-enzyme Q10), dark leafy greens, legumes, beans, soy, whole grains, water (6-8 glasses/day), extra virgin olive oil, and fresh fruit.

TOXIC EYE: Toxins play a more important role in eye diseases than is usually realized. The avoidance and elimination of pro-oxidant foods, toxic chemicals and heavy metals should be an integral part of promoting healthy eye care. Over exposure to air pollutants, pesticides, toxic medications, heavy metals, nicotine and tars, excessive alcohol, monosodium glutamate, aspartame cause oxidative stress, inflammation and ischemia. Avoidance is essential to good eye health.

INTERNAL DISEASES: Natural prevention and treatment measures should be considered over or complimentary to a quick fix of potentially adverse medications and invasive surgery.

Cataract: avoid excess sunlight, trauma, diabetes, adverse medications, smoking, junk food diet; take antioxidants, fresh fruit, spinach, broccoli, bilberry, blueberries, organic milk (glutathione), Brazil nuts (selenium), green tea, apples (quercetin), curry (turmeric), and omega-3 fish oil.

Glaucoma: exercise regularly: multivitamin with C, B1, B12, selenium, chromium, magnesium, beta-carotene(Vitamin A),; *Ginkgo biloba*.

Macular degeneration: avoid sun exposure, smoking, toxins, junk food,; take multivitamin with A, C, lutein, zeaxanthin, B vitamins(spinach, kale, collards), glutathione & taurine (onions, garlic, avocado, asparagus), minerals (zinc, chromium, copper, magnesium), omega-3 fish oil, red wine, dark chocolate, *Ginkgo biloba*, bilberry.

NUTRITION: Antioxidant nutrients with protective effects on ocular tissues prevent telomere shortening and may be useful for reducing the cumulative effects of oxidative stress. Omega-3 (EPA and DHA), lutein, zeaxanthin, zinc, selenium, turmeric, ginger, coenzymeQ10, green tea, quercetin, foods with carotenoids, bioflavonoids, isoflavones, polyphenols, garlic, dark leafy greens, berries, spices and culinary herb have all been researched and found to have beneficial effects on ocular tissues and their actions.

Nutritional Supplements For Ocular Tissues

Antioxidants: Vitamin A (retinol): dry eye mucin tear film, maculopathy

Vitamin C : healing, cataracts, diabetic retinopathy

Vitamin E: cataracts

Carotenoids (lutein, zeaxanthin): cataracts, retinal pigment epitheliopathy, maculopathy

Zinc: maculopathy
Selenium: cataract, cell membrane protection
Omega-3 fish oil: healing, DNA repair
Vitamin B6: aqueous tears, prostaglandin E1 synthesis

BOTANICALS: The most widely used, effective, evidence-based botanicals for eye care are bilberry, *Ginkgo biloba*, extracts of grapeseed and pinebark, saffron, and consumption of mixed vegetables. Many show antioxidant, anti-inflammation, antimicrobial, antiviral, astringent and circulation regulatory activities. For inflammation/infection control, goldenseal, borage, chamomile, and chrysanthemum are recommended. For cataracts, grapeseed extract, antioxidants with vitamin C, broccoli, ginger and turmeric have shown some effect. For pain and swelling of ocular tissues, : boswellia, ginger, turmeric, and willow bark are effective.

EXERCISE benefits the eyes by increasing chorioretinal blood flow, decreasing intraocular pressure, reducing the risk of cardiovascular disease, diabetes, hypertension, autoimmune and neurodegenerative diseases, regulating the immune system to reduce harmful inflammation and removing toxins through elimination.

STRESS releases cortisol which can lead to ocular tissue damage through peroxidation and reduction in immune system function. Therapeutic control can be achieved through breathing techniques and basic calming strategies. Botanicals and supplements with stress reducing properties include eleuthero root, rhodiola rosea, ashwagandha, cordyceps, passionflower, chamomile, skull cap, valerian, cowslip, coenzyme Q10, kava kava, and magnesium/calcium balance.

ENERGY MEDICINE involves using the properties of light, sound, touch and magnetic therapies for pain and stress reduction. They may benefit skin diseases, neonatal jaundice, emotional disorders, and age-related macular degeneration through mechanisms involving regulation of hormonal, biochemical and immunological responses, especially when the long term use of steroids and /or toxic drugs are contraindicated.

TRADITIONAL CHINESE & AYURVEDIC MEDICINE therapies of acupuncture, moxibustion, diets, exercises, and herbs are useful as adjuncts to conventional therapy especially for pain relief. The herbs are effective in blood cleansing, liver, gall bladder and kidney regulation, jaundice, dry eyes, and anxiety and depression in relation to insomnia.

HOMEOPATHY is non-toxic and may be effective in the treatment of some acute and chronic conditions like cataracts, glaucoma, stress control, inflammation-related conjunctivitis, uveitis, chorioretinitis and autoimmune diseases.

Some uses of homeopathic preparations for the eyes:
Lids: ledum, arsenicum
Conjunctivitis with discharge: rhus toxicodendrum, mercurius
Conjunctivitis redness with inflammation external: belladonna, pulsatilla,
aconite, euphrasia, sabadilla, ferrum phosphoricum, sulphur
Iritis redness with inflammation internal: gelsemium

Hyphema: hamamelis
Cataract: causticum, casticum, conium, calcarea flourica, silicea
Glaucoma: opium, cocaine muriate, spigella, aconitum napellus
Retinitis: phosphorus
Asthenopia: ruta graveolens

Complimentary Medical Therapies With Positive Evidence-Based Studies:

1. Acupuncture
2. Alexander technique
3. Aromatherapy
4. Autogenic therapy
5. Ayurvedic medicine
6. Biofeedback
7. Color therapy
8. Herbal medicine
9. Homeopathy
10. Hypnosis
11. Magnet therapy
12. Massage
13. Meditation
14. Naturopathy

About the Authors

The environment in which I was raised and still reside, provided my first introduction to natural health care. Traditional folk medicine in the Caribbean region is still widespread and those knowledgeable in its use are well respected and sought out. Despite our modernization during the 1960s when the pharmacy displaced the apothecary, attempts to push traditional medicine into the background were in vain.

Throughout medical school on the mainland, my interest in traditional medicine became stronger as applied biochemistry and physiology mixed easily with psychiatry and pathology and began to reveal the interrelationships of the human body, the mind, and the environment. I was fortunate to have attended Howard University in Washington, DC, which maintained strong connections in Native American and African American medicine due in part to its proximity to the Chesapeake Bay area and the fringes of the South. Upon returning to the islands and opening a practice in ophthalmology, a large number of my patients were eager and willing to discuss, question and exchange knowledge of the use of local herbals and traditional mores. Patients love to share their experiences and knowledge with someone who listens with sincere interest and doesn't dismiss their views but offers them options. "Sometimes it works and sometimes it doesn't, but here is how and why."

By 1986, having collected as many stories and anecdotes as a shoebox could hold, I published a small volume of colloquial terms, sayings, and remedies, entitled *Medical Terminology of the Eastern Caribbean.* Its intent was to preserve our rapidly disappearing cultural influence of health care. It is still generating interest and remains a local favorite.

In the 1990s, I became interested in French *ethnobotany* and had the opportunity to visit museums and medicinal gardens in Paris and Geneva. In 2005, I enrolled in the program in integrative medicine directed by Dr. Andrew Weil and the fine staff at the University of Arizona in Tucson. This program successfully highlighted the concept of well-being in health and contributed to a more complete picture of what health care should be. It set the stage for the continuous pursuit of the comprehensive treatment of the patient as a whole person and not just a statistic or body part.

Integrative Medicine is:

> "An approach to medicine that makes use of the best available evidence based therapies taking into account the whole person including all aspects of lifestyle."
>
> Andrew Weil, MD

In 2008, after successfully completing a two-year Master Herbalist certificate, which provided the tools to investigate and utilize the active parts of botanicals in health care, I was able to apply to grow and create blends of teas to be used as dietary aids for medical conditions by paying close attention to the chemical constituents of the plants and their specific actions. With this came the mountain farm in Puerto Rico where these plants flourish.

The doctors of the 20th century thrived on new technology; this era brought with it new methods of measurement, treatment, and reimbursement. The challenge now to 21st century doctors is to expand technology to incorporate a more clinical acumen that focuses more on life experiences, patient-doctor relationships, outcome expectations and broader treatment plans which include holistic options. More attention needs to be paid to quality of life. We need to temper our obsession with new technology and consider what it is we are doing in the field of medicine. What are we trying to accomplish? What is the definitive goal? I hope that this book offers some insight and stimulates discussion into topics other than just new technology.

Alfred L. Anduze, MD
Saluan Farm Health & Wellness Center
Maricao, Puerto Rico

My life as a physician (forty-two years) in academic, (Howard University Medicine and Faculty, University of Illinois Residency, Bascom Palmer Eye Institute Fellowship), rural, and Middle East Ophthalmic care has provided a continuum of change in eye diseases and their care through a Western medicine prism. Through this somewhat skewed view, I have come to recognize that the dictum: "If it is new, it is not true; and if it is true, it is not new!" applies to both rural and urban venues.

Consider primary open-angle glaucoma (POAG) as a leading cause of blindness in the USA and maybe the leading cause of blindness in people of African descent. The Western medicine approach is to attack the surrogate risk (increase intraocular pressure) by any means close-by, handy or procedure driven for monetary gain! There are six broad classes of topical pressure-lowering ophthalmic drops, numerous laser therapeutic approaches, and a vast array of surgical procedures. Cryo and thermal ablation procedures have come and gone.

These and other costly and usually ineffective therapies (in pigmented people) are not infrequently harmful. Experience has shown me that end-organ damage (viz. preservation of the optic nerves with confirmatory visual field evidence) is rare to nonexistent.

Numerous other ophthalmic disorders (viz. pterygium, keratomalacia, pseudotumor cerebri, toxic optic neuropathies, and early stages of diabetic retinal disorders) are best treated by known preventive modalities. It is our goal to inform our readers and thereby their patients that many sight-saving practices are present in common plants, foods, and life behaviorial changes. Simply consider the IOP-lowering effects of smoked (inhaled) Cannabis sativa L. to treat the surrogate risk of raised IOP in the glaucomas, or the spice turmeric to reduce systemic inflammation thereby reducing dementia and arthritis. Look around—God gave us numerous therapeutic interventions for all our present-day disorders before he gave us lasers.

John C. Merritt, MD
Prevention for the People, Inc.
Clinton, NC, 28328 USA